Traditional Chinese Treatment for Psychogenic and Neurogenic Diseases

Chief-Editor: Hou Jinglun

Editors: Zhao Xin

Geng Chun'e

Li Guohua

Academy Press [Xue Yuan]

First Edition 1996

ISBN 7 - 5077 - 1182 - X/R· 207

Traditional Chinese Treatment for Psychogenic and Neurogenic Diseases
Chief - Editor: Hou Jinglun
Editors: Zhao Xin   Li Guohua
Published by
Academy Press [Xue Yuan]
11 Wanshoulu Xijie, Beijing 100036, China

Distributed by
China International Book Trading Corporation
35 Chegongzhuang Xilu, Beijing 100044, China
P. O. Box 399, Beijing, China

Printed in the People' s Republic of China

Introduction to Collections
of Traditional Chinese Medicine

Traditional Chinese Medince and Pharmacology (TCMP) has a long history. TCMP sumed up abundant clinical experience in the struggle against diseases. It has formed an integrated, unique and first of all, a scientific system of both theory and clincial practice. On the fundamental principle of "Zhengtiguannian" (Wholism) and "Bianzhenglunzhi" (Treatment of the same disease with different therapies), TCM treatment is effective for various kinds of diseases with few side-effect taken. At present, a great upsurge in learning, practising and studying TCM is just in the accendant. For the benefit of people of all countries, we compiled this series of "Collections of Traditional Chinese Medicine" in order to promote the spread of TCM all over the world. In these books, we introduced comprehensively TCM treatment of commonly encountered diseases and therapies such as drug therapy, acupuncture and moxibustion, Qigong, massage, dietic therapy, etc. are suggested accordingly. This series is the best for those foreign friends who want to learn and master TCM.

May everyone of all nations enjoy a healthy life!

Chief-Editor

CONTENTS

Chapter One
Peripheral Facial Paralysis
(Bell's palsy)

Bell's palsy is a paralysis of one side of the face, is facial paralysis which occurs suddenly and mostly after exposure to cold wind or trauma. It may occur at any age but is slightly more common in the age group from 20 to 50. 85 – 90% of the patients get recovered spontaneously. In traditional Chinese medicine, the onset of the illness is thought to be due to derangement of qi and blood and malnutrition of the channels caused by invasion of the channels and collaterals in the facial region by pathogenic wind-cold or phlegm. If falls into the category of "zhen zhong feng", "kou yan wai xie" or "diao xian feng" (deviation of the eye and mouth) in traditional Chinese medicine.

I. MAIN POINTS OF DIAGNOSIS

1. It often occurs in autumn and winter or between spring and summer, mostly in the middle-aged. The disease usually attacks one side of the face.

2. The diagnosis is based on the symptoms, but most rule out cerebrovascular accidents (strokes) and intracranial tumors. The peripheral facial paralysis patients are specially unable to frown and raise the eyebrow, close the eye of the paralyzed side. The intracranial tumors can be ruled out on X-ray examination.

3. The attack comes all of a sudden. At the beginning the patient feels numb at one side of the face, pain around the ear and tenderness in the mastoidal region. Then the mouth becomes wry, the nasolabial groove no longer seen and the facio-buccal region relaxed and strengthless. It's impossible to have the cheeks blown up. The eyeballs are still exposed when the eyes are shut. It's dif-

ficult to frown and speak. Salivation comes down from the corners of the mouth. The sense of taste is lost but the sense of hearing is hypersensitive. There may be pain in the mastoid region or headache.

II. TREATMENT OF COMMON SYNDROMES

1. Internal Treatment
1) The Early Stage
Main Symptoms and Signs: The onset is sudden and the duration is short. The mouth and eyes become wry. the eyeballs can always be seen as the eyes can not be closed entirely. There is difficulty in frowning. The accompanying symptoms and signs are headache, discomfort or low fever, red tongue with thin and white fur, and taut and thready pulse.

Therapeutic Principles: Dispelling pathogenic wind and removing obstruction from the channels.

Recipe: Yang-clearing Decoction with Additional Ingredients

Radix Astragali seu Hedysari	15 g
Radix Angelicae Sinensis	15 g
Fructus Tribuli	15 g
Rhizoma Cimicifugae	9 g
Flos Carthami	9 g
Cortex Phellodendri	9 g
Ramulus Cinnamomi	9 g
Lignum Sappan	9 g
Radix Ledebouriellae	9 g
Periostracum Cicadae	9 g
Radix Puerariae	30 g
Radix Glycyrrhizae	6 g

All the above drugs are to be decocted in water for oral administration.
2) The Late Stage
Main Symptoms and Signs: The course of the disease is protracted. The

mouth and the eyes become wry. No wrinkles can

be seen on the forehead. The patient has reddish tongue with petechiae on it, thin and white fur, and thready and feeble pulse.

Therapeutic Principles: Promoting qi flow and blood circulation, removing phlegm and clearing away obstruction from the channels.

Recipe: Powder for Treating Wry-Mouth, compounded with Decoction Invigorating Yang for Recuperation

Rhizoma Typhonii	6 g
Scorpio	9 g
Bombyx Batryticatus	9 g
Semen Persicae	9 g
Flos Carthami	9 g
Lumbricus	9 g
Radix Astragali seu Hedysari	30 g
Radix Angelicae Sinensis	15 g
Rhizoma Ligustici Chuanxiong	15 g
Radix Paeoniae Rubra	15 g

All the above drugs are to be decocted in water for oral administration.

For those running low fever, add 30 grams of isatis root and 30 grams of honeysuckle flower. For those with restlessness due to deficiency and palpitation, add 18 grams of prepared rehmannia root and 18 grams of prepared fleece-flower root and suffocation in the chest and stomach and who are fat and have much sputum, add 6 grams of arisaema with bile and 9 grams of pinellia tuber.

Another herb therapy is Zhi Jing San Jia Jian

Recipe	
Scorpion	2.5 g
Fangfeng	13 g
Larvia of silkworm of rehmannia	10 g
Baifuzi	10 g
Milk veteh	30 g
Chinese angelica	15 g
Unpeeled root of herbaceous peony	15 g

Chuanxiong	15 g
Peach Kernel	15 g
Safflower	12 g

.   All the above herbs make a dose and six to ten doses are prescribed with one dose daily. Each dose is simmered twice and then the broth of each mixed, half of the mixed broth each time, twice a day.

2. External Treatment

1) Apply Adhesive Plaster on the Acupoints: Dust 0.5 to 1 gram of the powder of Semen Strychni onto a plaster and then apply the plaster on the acupoint of Taiyang(EX-HN5), Xiaguan(ST7) and Jiache(ST6) of the affected side (more applicable to the regions with tenderness). Change the plaster every 3 days. If blisters appear on the administered part, extract its fluid after disinfection. Then the blisters will get cured spontaneously.

2) Smear the Blood of Eel onto the Affected Region: Smear fresh blood of eel onto the buccal skin of the affected side, and hold the mouth angle of the affected side with a metal hook so as to help cure the facial paralysis. This is to be done once a day.

3) Do Local Massage on the Affected Region: Several times a day.

4) Acupuncture Therapy

Points: Yifeng(SJ17), Dicang(ST4), Jiache(ST6), Yangbai(GB14), Taiyang(EX-HN5), Hegu(LI4), Quanliao(SI18) and Xiaguan(ST7).

Method: 3 to 5 of the above points are selected for each treatment and the therapy is given once daily. Dicang(ST4) and Jiache(ST6) are punctured together with one needle inserted horizontally from Dicang(ST4) to Jiache(ST6). The following points can also be added to the formula according to the symptoms: Fengchi(GB20) for headache; Fenglong(ST40) for profuse sputum; Cuanzhu(BL2) and Sizhukong(SJ23) for difficulty in frowning and raising the eyebrow; Cuanzhu(BL2), Jingming(BL1), Tongziliao(BL15), Yuyao(EX-HN4) and Sizhukong(SJ23) for incomplete closing of the eyelids; Yingxiang(LI20) for difficulty in sniffing; Shuigou(RN26) for deviation of the philtrum; Juliao(ST3) for inability to show the teeth; Tinghui(GB2) for tinnitus and deafness; Wangu(SI4) for tenderness at the mastoid region; and Taichong(LR3) for twitching of the eyelid and the mouth.

5) Electro-acupuncture Therapy

Main Points: Qianzheng(an extra-point) and Yifeng(SJ17).

Auxiliary Points: Yangbai(GB14), Taiyang(EX-HN5) and Dicang(ST4).

Method: One of the main points and two or three of the auxiliary points are prescribed each time. The main point is connected to the negative pole of the electro-acupuncture machine, and the auxiliary points to the positive pole. The frequency is adjusted to 20 to 30 times per minute with an output which can just cause the muscular twitch on the affected side. The treatment lasts for 15 minutes and is repeated once every other day. Ten times consisted of one course.

The patient can be assured that recovery usually occurs in 2 to 8 weeks (or up to one to two years in older patients). In the vast majority of cases, partial or complete recovery occurs. When recovery is partial, contractures may develop on the paralyzed side. Recurrence on the same or the opposite side is occasionally reported. Acupuncture therapy is very effective for this condition.

III. THERAPEUTIC METHODS BY PRACTISING QIGONG

1. Self-Treatment by Practising Qigong

1) Basic Maneuvers

It is advisable to practise Head and Face Qigong.

2) Auxiliary Maneuvers

Those shedding tears ought to lay emphasis on kneading Yangbai(GB14), Sibai(ST2), and Tongziliao(GB1).

At the onset stage, the pressing and kneading manipulations applied locally should be light; as for those with a long course of disease, the manipulations should be heavier.

2. External Qi Therapy

1) Basic Maneuvers

(1) Press and knead the acupoints Yangbai (GB14), Chengqi (ST1), Sizhukong(SJ23), Tongziliao(GB1), Tinggong(SI19), Yifeng(SJ17), Quanliao(SI18), Yingxiang(LI20), Jiache(ST6), Fengchi(GB20) and Hegu(LI4).

(2) Apply the flat-palm form, use the pushing, pulling and leading manipulations to emit qi onto the unilateral paralyzed face, conduct the channel qi from front to back and along the Large Intestine Meridian to the terminals of the upper extremities.

2) Auxiliary Maneuvers

In the anaphase of the paralysis, the additional application of the vibrating and quivering manipulation is advised to provoke the channel qi.

IV. TREATMENT BY CHINESE MASSAGE

There will be gradual recovery in one or two weeks after its onset. Manipulation of massage may help the recovery of facial nerves and muscular function and reduce sequelae. During the treatment, stimulus of cold to the face and head should be avoided and the patient should knead the face frequently for enhancing the effectiveness.

1. Manipulation: Pushing with one-finger meditation, digital-pressing, pressing, grasping and kneading.

2. Location of Points: Hegu(LI4), Quchi(LI11), Xiaguan(ST7), Jiache (ST6), Yifeng(SJ17), Taiyang(EX-HN5), Jingming(BL1), Sibai(ST2), Yingxiang(LI20), Shuigou(DU26) and Dicang(ST4).

3. Operation

1) The doctor stands in front and to the side of the sitting patient and holds the posterolateral part of the head with one hand. Using one-finger meditation pushing or thumb-pressing- kneading, the doctor pushes with the other hand repeatedly from Yintang(EX-HN3) along the supercilliary of the affected side to Taiyang(EX-HN5) for 2 or 3 times first; then pushes repeatedly from Yintang (EX-HN3) upwards by way of Shenting(DU24) to Baihui(DU20) also for 2 or 3 times; finally, pushes repeatedly from the middle of the forehead via Yangbai (GB14) of the affected part to Taiyang(EX-HN5) for 2 or 3 times.

2) After that, in the above-mentioned way, the doctor pushes downwards repeatedly from Yintang(EX-HN3) by way of Jingming(BL1) of the affected

side, along the side of the nose up to Yingxiang(LI20) for 2 or 3 times. Then the doctor pushes from Yingxiang(LI20), along the point of Sibai(ST2), Quan-liao(SI18), Xiaguan(ST7) and Jiache(ST6) passing the face, to Dicang(ST4) at the labial angle.

3) Still in the same way mentioned above, the operator pushes from Dicang (ST4) to Shuigou(DU26) circling the lips, by way of Chengjiang(RN24), and returns to the starting point. Then the operator pushes along the mandible to Ji-ache(ST6). Finally rub and scrub softly the affected side of the face with the palm till local warmth and heat are produced.

In the above-mentioned operations, the movement of the hand should pass at every point with a bit more strength exerted and some stimulating manipulations such as digit-pressing used in combination.

4) The doctor stands to the side of the patient and, with one hand holding his forehead, grasps Fengchi(GB20) and the tendons of the back nape up and down repeatedly for three to five times, finally pushes the point Qiaogong for 30 times.

5) The doctor standing behind the patient, grasps Jianjing(GB21) with two hands and in an orderly way presses and kneads Quchi(LI11) and Hegu(LI4).

4. Course of Treatment: Once a day, six days for one course with an inter-val of 3 days between two courses.

Chapter Two
Headache

Headache is a kind of clinically common-subjective symptom. It can be accompanied by various kinds of acute and chronic diseases. This section will mainly discuss some symptoms characterised mainly by headache.

I. CLINICAL MANIFESTATIONS

1. Headache due to Exopathy

1) Headache due to Pathogenic Wind-Cold Pathogen: frequent headache, pain extending to the nape and back, aversion to cold and wind, joy for head-binding, no thirst, thin and whitish tongue fur, floating and tense pulse.

2) Headache due to Pathogenic Wind-Heat: distension and pain in the head, fever, aversion to wind, thirst with desire to drink, dark urine, reddened tongue with thin and yellow fur, floating and rapid pulse.

3) Headache due to Pathogenic Summer-Heat and Dampness: strong binding pain in the head, lassitude of limbs, poor appetite, fullness in the epigastric region, fever, sweating, dysphoria, thirst, greasy fur and slippery pulse.

2. Headache due to Internal Injury

1) Headache due to Abnormal Ascending of Liver-Yang: headache with intermittent dizziness, dysphoria, irritability, insomnia, bitter taste, reddened tongue with thin and yellow fur, taut and forceful pulse.

2) Headache due to Stagnation of Phlegm: Headache with dizziness, fullness in the epigastric region, vomiting, abundant expectoration, whitish and greasy fur, slippery or taut and slippery pulse.

3) Headache due to Deficiency of Blood: Headache and dizziness which be-

come intense with slight labour, weakness, dysphoria, palpitation, shortness of breath, pale complexion, pale tongue with thin and whitish fur, thready and feeble pulse.

4) Headache due to Deficiency of Kidney: Headache with a sensation of emptiness inside the head, dizziness, weakness and lassitude in the loin and legs, emission, leucorrhagia, tinnitus, insomnia, reddened tongue with little fur, thready and feeble pulse.

II. DIFFERENTIATION

1. Headache due to Invasion of Pathogenic Wind into the Channels and Collaterals: Headache occurs often, especially on exposure to wind. The pain may extend to the nape of the neck and back regions. Thin and white tongue coating, floating pulse.

2. Headache due to Upsurge of Liver-Yang: headache, distension of the head, irritability, hot temper, dizziness, blurring of vision, red tongue with thin and yellow coating, taut and rapid pulse.

3. Headache due to Deficiency of both Qi and Blood: Lingering headache, dizziness, blurring of vision, lassitude, lustreless face, pale tongue with thin and white coating, thin and weak pulse.

III. TREATMENT BY ACUPUNCTURE

1. Body Acupuncture

Prescription: Baihui(DU20), Taiyang(EX-HN5) and Hegu(LI4).

Supplementary Points: In the treatment of headache due to invasion of pathogenic wind into channels and collaterals, supplementary points should be selected according to the channel and collateral in which the pain is located. For example, for frontal headache, Yintang(EX-HN3), Shangxing(DU23) and Neiting(ST44); for temporal headache, Waiguan(SJ5) and Zulingqi(GB41); for parietal headache, Houxi(SI3), Taichong(LR3) and Zhiyin(BL67); for occipital headache, Fengchi(GB20), Kunlun(BL60). In the treatment of headache due to upsurge of liver-yang, Fengchi(GB20), Xiaxi(GB43) and Xingjian(LR2) are added. In the treatment of headache due to deficiency of both qi and blood, Qihai(RN6), Zusanli(ST36), Pishu(BL20) and Shenshu(BL23) are added.

Method: Use the filiform needles to puncture the points with reinforcing method and moxibustion, for headache due to deficiency of both qi and blood, and with the reducing method or even movement for the other two types of headache.

2. Auricular Acupuncture

Prescription: Pt. occiput, Pt. Forehead, Pt. Brain, Pt. Shenmen, Pt. Kidney and Pt. Spleen

Method: Select 2-3 points for each treatment. Retain the needles for 30 minutes. The auricular-seed-pressing therapy may also be used.

IV. THERAPEUTIC METHODS
BY PRACTISING QIGONG

1. Self-Treatment by Practising Qigong.

1) Basic Maneuvers

It is advisable to practise Relaxation Qigong and Head and Face Qigong.

2) Auxiliary Maneuvers

(1) Shaoyang headache: Lay particular stress on relaxing from the bilateral sides of the head along the Triple Warmer Meridian of Hand-Shaoyang and Gall Bladder Meridian of Foot- Shaoyang to the upper and lower limbs successively.

(2) Taiyang headache: Lay particular emphasis on relaxing from the vertex along the Small Intestine Meridian of Hand-Taiyang and Urinary Bladder Meridian of Foot-Taiyang to the upper and lower limbs successively.

(3) Jueyin headache: Lay particular emphasis on relaxing from the vertex along the Liver Meridian of Foot-Jueyin to the lower limbs successively.

(4) Yangming headache: Lay particular emphasis on relaxing from the forehead along the Large Intestine Meridian of Hand-Yangming and the Stomach Meridian of Foot-Yangming to the upper and lower limbs successively.

(5) Deficiency of qi and blood: It is advisable to practise Inner-Nourishing Qigong and Roborant Qigong.

2. External Qi Therapy

1) Basic Maneuvers

(1) Press and knead Yintang(EX-HN3), Taiyang(EX-HN5), Baihui (DU20), Fengfu(DU16), Fengchi(GB20), Hanyan(GB4), Quchi(LI11) and Hegu(LI4).

(2) Apply the flat-palm form, use the pushing pulling and leading manipulations to emit qi onto the headache region, and conduct qi along the Ren Channel to Guanyuan(RN4).

2) Auxiliary Maneuvers

(1) Shaoyang headache: Apply the flat-palm form, use the pulling and leading manipulations to emit qi onto Shuaigu(GB8), Jiaosun(SJ20) and Hanyan (GB4), and conduct the channel qi along the Triple Warmer Meridian of Hand-Shaoyang and the Gall Bladder Meridian of Foot-Shaoyang.

(2) Taiyang headache: Apply the flat-palm form, use the pushing and leading manipulations to emit qi onto Quchi(LI11) and Tianzhu(BL10), and conduct the channel qi along the Channels of Hand-and Foot-Taiyang to the upper and lower limbs.

(3) Jueyin headache: Apply the flat-palm form, use the pulling and rotating manipulations to rotate rightward to conduct qi, and conduct the channel qi along the Gall Bladder Meridian to the lower limbs.

(4) Yangming headache: Apply the flat-palm form, use the pulling and leading manipulations to emit qi onto Taiyang(EX-HN5), Touwei(ST8) and Yintang(EX-HN3), and conduct the channel qi along the Channels of Hand- and Foot-Yangming to the upper and lower limbs.

(5) Deficiency of qi and blood: Apply the flat-palm form, use the pushing and leading manipulations to emit qi onto Pishu (BL20), Geshu (BL17),

Danzhong(RN17), Zhongwan(RN12) and Guanyuan(RN4).

V. TREATMENT BY CHINESE MASSAGE

Massage has a great remitting effect on headache, especially on headache due to cold, migraine and muscular contraction, headache.

1. Manipulation: Pushing with one-finger meditation, lifting-grasping, wiping, flat-pushing, pressing-kneading, etc..

2. Prescription of Points: Yintang(EX-HN3), Taiyang(EX-HN5), Jingming(BL1), Fengchi(GB20), Feishu(BL13), Ganshu(BL18) and Shenshu(BL23).

3. Operation

1) The patient is in a sitting position. The doctor, sitting behind the patient, lift-grasps the cervical point with the thumb and the four fingers from below to above 30 – 50 times.

2) Wipe the forehead and supercilliary arch in two directions, digital pressing Jingming(BL1), whip Yingxiang(LI20), Shuigou(DU26) and Chengjiang (RN24) in two directions for 3 – 5 times respectively. This should be repeated 3 times.

3) Sweep the temple for 30 to 50 times.

4) Grasping with the five fingers along the five channels of Du, Taiyang and Shaoyin from front to back. This should be repeated for 3 – 5 times.

5) Flat-push the chest and back till they become penetratedly hot; grasp Jianjing(GB21), the upper arms, forearms; foulage-shake the upper limbs; rotate the shoulders forwards and backwards for 3 circles respectively.

4. Modification of Manipulation According to Different Syndromes

1) Headache due to Wind-Cold Pathogen: Also press and knead Feishu (BL13) and Dazhu(BL11); straightly scrub the Urinary Bladder Meridian at the two sides of the spine till they become penetratedly hot and slightly sweating. Press and knead Quchi(LI11) and Hegu(LI4) till they become aching and dis-

tending.

2) Headache due to Wind-Heat Pathogen: Additionally, push Dazhui (DU14) with one-finger meditation for 3 - 5 minutes; pat and hit the Urinary Bladder Meridian at the two sides of the spine till the skin becomes reddish.

3) Headache due to Pathogenic Summer-Heat: Also pat and hit the Urinary Bladder Meridian at the two sides till the skin becomes reddish, and pinch Yintang(EX-HN3) and nuchal region till there appears slight blood stasis in the skin.

4) The Liver-Yang Headache: In addition, push Qiaogong, sweep the temple, obliquely-push two costal regions, press-knead Ganshu (BL18), Yanglingquan(GB34) and Taichong(LR3).

5) Headache due to Stagnation of Phlegm: Also press-knead Pishu(BL20), Weishu(BL21), Zusanli(ST36) and Fenglong(ST40), rub the abdomen, push Zhongwan(RN12) and Qihai(RN6) with one-finger meditation.

6) Headache due to Deficiency of Blood: Additionally pinch the spine for 3 to 5 times, press-knead Xinshu(BL15), Geshu(BL17) and Zusanli(ST36), rub the abdomen, push Zhongwan(RN12) and Qihai(RN6) with one-finger meditation.

7) Headache due to Kidney Deficiency: Also flat-push the lumbosacral portion, press-knead Shenshu(BL23) and Mingmen(DU4); rub the abdomen, push Qihai(RN6) and Guanyuan(RN4) with one-finger meditation.

5. Course of Treatment: Once a day, 3 times as one course for headache due to exopathy and 10 times as one course for the headache due to internal injury.

Chapter Three
Neurosis

Neurosis is caused by long-term mental stress which results in imbalance of excito-inhibitory process of cerebral cortex. The patients get excited or fatigue easily, and are frequently accompanied with various forms of somatic discomfort. It is more common in middle-aged females. In traditional Chinese medicine, this disease is categorized as "bu mei" (insomnia), "xin ji" (palpitation), "jian wang" (amnesia), "xuan yun" (dizziness), "tou tong" (headache), "xu sun" (consumptive disease), "yu zheng" (melancholia), "yi jing" (emission), "yang wei" (impotence), "zang zao" (hysteria), etc..

I. MAIN POINTS OF DIAGNOSIS

1. There is a history of mental conflict, or a long period of mental stress.

2. Major Clinical Manifestations

(1) Dyssomnia and reduced cerebral functions such as insomnia, dreaminess, waking up easily, distractibility and bad memory.

(2) The emotion is easy to be changed, accompanied with restlessness, hypersensitivity, poor tolerance to the sound and light.

(3) Functional disorders of the viscera: The patients frequently complain of palpitation, abdominal distension, belching, anorexia, constipation, frequency of micturition, impotence, etc..

3. The organic diseases should be excluded after examinations of nervous and visceral functions.

II. DIFFERENTIATION AND
TREATMENT OF COMMON SYNDROMES

1. Stagnation of the Liver-qi

Main Symptoms and Signs: Emotional depression, doubting mania, anxiety, vertigo, blurring of vision, fullness in the abdomen, eructation, anorexia, feeling of oppression in the chest, hypochondriac pain, irregular menstruation, reddish tongue with whitish fur, taut and thready pulse.

Therapeutic Principle: Dispersing depressed liver-qi to relieve emotional depression.

Recipe: Modified Bupleurum Powder for Relieving Liver-qi

Radix Bupleuri	10 g
Rhizoma Cyperi	10 g
Radix Curcumae	10 g
Fructus Aurantii	10 g
Radix Paeoniae Alba	10 g
Flos Albiziae	10 g
Radix Salviae Miltiorrhizae	10 g
Rhizoma Pinelliae	10 g
Pericarpium Citri Reticulatae	10 g

All the above drugs are to be decocted in water for oral administration.

In addition, the recipe should include 10 grams of both medicated leaven (Massa Fermentata Medicinalis) and membrane of chicken's gizzard (Endothelium Corneum Gigeriae Galli) if the case is with indigestion; 12 grams of pinellia tuber (Rhizoma Pinelliae) for the case with eructation and oppressed sensation in the chest; 10 grams of moutan bark (Cortex Moutan Radicis) and 10 grams of capejasmine (Fructus Gardeniae) when a disorder is ascribed to the fire-transmission due to stagnation of qi marked by bitter taste in the mouth, restlessness, headache, conjunctival congestion, red tongue with yellow fur, and taut rapid pulse; 10 grams of chrysanthemum (Flos Chrysanthemi) and 15 grams of uncaria stem with hooks (Ramulus Uncariae cum Uncis) to treat such symptoms as dizziness and feeling of fullness in the head.

Patent Medicine: Ease Pill (Xiao yao wan). Take 6 g each time, 3 times a day.

2. Hyperactivity of Fire due to Yin Deficiency

Main Symptoms and Signs: Anxiety, insomnia, dizziness, tinnitus, feverish sensation in the palms and soles, dry mouth with a few saliva, nocturnal emission, spermatorrhoea, premature ejaculation, palpitation, amnesia, soreness of waist, red tongue with yellowish fur, thready and rapid pulse.

Therapeutic Principle: Nourishing yin to clear away pathogenic fire.

Recipe: Modified prescriptions of Decoction of Coptis and Donkey-hide Gelatin and Heart-tonifying Bolus

Radix Rehmanniae	15 g
Radix Angelicae Sinensis	10 g
Radix Paeoniae Alba	10 g
Radix Ophiopogonis	10 g
Rhizoma Coptidis	6 g
Semen Ziziphi Spinosae	12 g
Caulis Polygoni Multifori	30 g
Fructus Schisandrae	10 g
Poria cum Ligno Hospite	10 g
Radix Salviae Miltiorrhizae	10 g
Radix Glycyrrhizae Praeparata	6 g
Colla Corii Asini	10 g

All the above drugs are to be decocted in water for oral administration. Besides, donkey-hide gelatin is melted with the decoction for oral use.

If the patient is extremely disturbed by insomnia, 30 grams of raw fossil fragments (Os Draconis) and 30 grams of oyster shell (Concha Ostreae) ought to be administered. If deficiency of the liver-yin and kidney-yin is remarkable with symptoms of soreness and weakness of the loins and knees, 20 grams of prepared rehmannia root (Radix Rehmanniae Praeparata) and 12 grams of wolfberry fruit (Fructus Lycii) be included. When a disorder is caused by insufficiency of the kidney-yang manifested as spermatorrhea, impotence, premature ejaculation, aversion to cold, cold limbs, listlessness, pale tongue, weak and deep pulse, the treatment should be aimed at tonifying the kidney-yang. The preferred recipe is modified Kidney-yang-reinforcing Bolus. The compositions are: prepared rehmannia root (Radix Rehmanniae Praeparata) 20 g, Chinese yam (Rhizoma Dioscoreae) 12 g, wolfberry fruit (Fructus Lycii) 12 g, fruit of medicinal cornel (Fructus Corni) 12 g, dodder seed (Semen Cuscutae) 12 g, morinda root (Radix Morindae) 12 g, antler glue (Colla Cornu Cervi) 10 g (melted in boiling water for oral administration with the decoction), red raspberry (Fructus Rubi) 10 g, prepared aconite root (Radix Aconiti Praeparata) 6 g, epimedium (Herba Epimedii) 10 g, curculigo rhizome (Rhizoma Curculiginis) 10 g. All the above drugs are to be decocted in water for oral administration.

Patent Medicine: Cardiotonic Bolus (Heart-tonifying bolus, tian wang bu xin dan). Take 9 g each time, twice a day.

3. Deficiency of the Heart and Spleen

Main Symptoms and Signs: Dreaminess and being easy to wake, palpitation, amnesia, fatigue and weakness, anorexia, sallow complexion, pale tongue with thin whitish fur, thready and weak pulse.

Therapeutic Principle: Invigorating the heart and spleen.

Recipe: Modified Decoction for Invigorating the Spleen and Nourishing the Heart.

Radix Astragali seu Hedysari	15 g
Radix Codonopsis Pilosulae	12 g
Rhizoma Atractylodis Macrocephalae	10 g
Radix Angelicae Sinensis	10 g
Semen Ziziphi Spinosae	12 g
Radix Polygalae	10 g
Radix Aucklandiae	6 g
Radix Glycyrrhizae Praeparata	3 g

All the above drugs are to be decocted in water for oral administration.

If the patient is troubled by frequent insomnia, the recipe should include schisandra fruit (Fructus Schisandrae) 10 g, fleeceflower stem (Caulis Polygoni Multiflori) 30 g, or arborvitae seed (Semen Biotae) 10 g, raw fossil fragments (Os Draconis) 20 g, oyster shell (Concha Ostreae) 20 g, and if the patient complains of anorexia, 10 grams of membrane of chicken's gizzard (Endothelium

Corneum Gigeriae Galli). When a disorder is persistent depression resulting in impairment of the mind characterized by trance, dysphoria, sadness and melancholy and tending to cry, pale tongue with thin whitish fur, string-like and thready pulse, the treatment should be aimed at nourishing the heart to tranquillize the mind. Decoction of Licorice, Wheat and Chinese-Date with additional ingredients can be chosen for the case. It includes the following drugs:

Radix Glycyrrhizae Praeparata	10 g
Fructus Tritici Levis	30 g
Fructus Ziziphi Jujubae	10 pieces
Semen Ziziphi Spinosae	12 g
Semen Biotae	12 g
Flos Albiziae	15 g
Dens Draconis	20 g
Radix Curcumae	10 g

All the above drugs are to be decocted in water for oral administration.

4. Stagnation of Qi due to Phlegm Accumulation

Main Symptoms and Signs: Uncomfortable sensation of the throat, a foreign body sensation in the throat, hard to spit it out or to swallow it, chest distress, or accompanied by hypochondriac pain. Thin and greasy tongue coating, wiry and slippery pulse.

Therapeutic Principles: Resolve phlegm and regulate qi to alleviate mental depression.

Recipe

Pinellia tuber	9 g
magnolia bark	15 g
poria	15 g
perilla leaf	9 g
fresh ginger	9 g
nutgrass flatsedge rhizome	9 g
citron fruit	9 g
finger citron	9 g
inula flower	9 g
red ochre	30 g

Patent Medicine: Stagnation-Relieving Pill (Yueju Wan). Take 9 g each time, twice a day.

III. TREATMENT BY ACUPUNCTURE
AND MOXIBUSTION

1. Body Acupuncture

Main Points: Neiguan(PC6), Fenglong(ST40), Danzhong(RN17) and Xinshu(BL15).

Complementary Points: Ganshu (BL18), Zhongwan (RN12), Zusanli (ST36), Gongsun(SP4) and Taichong(LR3) are added for treating depression of qi in the liver; Zhigou(SJ6), Yanglingquan(GB34), Xingjian(LR2) and Xiaxi (GB43) for transformation of depressed qi into fire; Tiantu(RN22) and Taichong(LR3) for stagnation of phlegm and qi.

Method: Use filiform needles to puncture the points with even movement or reducing method.

2. Auricular Acupuncture

Prescribed Points: Shenmen, Occiput, Heart, Stomach and Brain.

Method: 2 or 3 points are selected for each treatment. The needles are twisted with moderate or strong stimulation and retained for 15 minutes. Throat and Esophagus are added to treat stagnation of phlegm and qi.

IV. THERAPEUTIC METHODS
BY PRACTISING QIGONG

1. Self-Treatment by Practising Qigong (1)

Stand relaxedly with both arms naturally hanging down with the palms facing downward and the five fingers of each hand slightly held up; press down with slight force and imagine qi to reach the palms and the fingertips for 3 times. Lift both hands to both sides in front of the chest with the palms facing forward, focus the mind on both palms, push the palms forward and then draw them back to the front of the chest. Stretch both hands levelly out to the left and right respectively, with the ten fingers pointing upward and the palms pushing vertically to the left and right respectively, with qi flowing to the front of the chest with the palms facing upward with the fingertips of one hand pointing at those of the other, focus the mind on both palms, then tun over the palms to face downward, and push them to the symphysis pubis. When qi flows to the lower Dantian, turn over the palms to face upward so as to hold and send qi to the middle Dantian. Do it this way for 3 times.

2. Self-Treatment by Practising Qigong (2)

1) Basic Maneuvers

It is advisable to practise Relaxation Qigong, Inner- Nourishing Qigong and Roborant Qigong.

2) Auxiliary Maneuvers

(1) Stagnation of the liver-qi: It is advisable to practise the methods of rubbing the chest and training qi with the word "xu" as well as soothing the liver and conducting qi in Regulating-Liver Qigong.

(2) Deficiency of the liver-yin and kidney-yin: It is advisable to practise Gathering Moon Cream Qigong, the methods of rubbing the abdomen to strengthen elixir and rubbing the abdomen to strengthen qi in Abdomen Qigong.

(3) Deficiency of the heart and the spleen: It is advisable to practise the methods of taking yellow qi and dredging the spleen and the stomach in Regulating-Spleen Qigong as well as the method of taking red qi in Regulating-Heart Qigong.

3. External Qi Therapy

1) Basic Maneuvers

(1) Press and knead Dazhui(DU14), Baihui(DU20) and Taiyang(EX-HN5), push and knead Hanyan(GB4) and Shuaigu(GB8), tip and knead Ganshu(BL18), Shenshu(BL23), Guanyuan(RN4) and Qihai(RN6).

(2) Apply the flat-palm form, use the vibrating manipulation to emit qi onto the acupoints Baihui(DU20), Dazhui(DU14), Zhongwan(RN12) and Guanyuan(RN4) for 12 or 24 breaths respectively.

(3) Apply the flat-palm form, use the pulling and leading manipulations to emit qi onto Touwei(ST8), Liangmen(ST21), Zusanli(ST36), Baihui(DU20), Zhongwan(RN12) and Guanyuan(RN4), and conduct the channel qi along the

Du Channel from Baihui(DU20) to Guanyuan(RN4), then conduct the channel qi along the Stomach Channel from touwei(ST8) to Zusanli(ST36).

2) Auxiliary Maneuvers

(1) Stagnation of liver-qi: Apply the flat-palm form, use the pulling and leading manipulations to conduct the channel qi from Qimen(LR14) along the Liver Meridian to the lower limbs.

(2) Deficiency of the liver-yin and kidney-yin: Apply the flat-palm form, use the pushing and vibrating manipulations to emit qi onto Ganshu(LR18), Shenshu(BL23) and Guanyuan(RN4).

(3) Deficiency of both the heart and the spleen: Apply the flat-palm form, use the pushing and quivering manipulations to emit qi onto the acupoints Xinshu(BL15), Pishu(BL20), Juque(RN14) and Zhongwan(RN12).

V. TREATMENT BY CHINESE MASSAGE

Massotherapy for this disease proves to be effective. During treatment, the patient should have a good rest and be free from worries and cares.

1. Manipulation: Pushing with one-finger meditation, kneading, flat-pushing, wiping, sweeping, grasping and rubbing.

2. Location of Points: Yintang(EX-HN3), Shenting(DU24), Jingming(BL1), Cuanzhu (BL20), Taiyang (EX-HN5), Jiaosun (SJ20), Fengchi(GB20), Jianjing(GB21), Zhongwan(RN12), Qihai(RN6), Guanyuan(RN4) and the Stream Points (Shu-Points) on the back.

3. Operation

1) The patient is in a sitting position. The doctor stands posterolateral to the patient, holding the patient's forehead with the palmar sides of the thumb, fore finger and middle finger of one hand, with the thumb and the two fingers grasping Fengchi(GB20) and the tendon of back nape from above to below for a dozen time, and pushing the left and right Qiaogong for 20 – 30 times respectively.

2) The doctor, standing in front of the sitting patient, separately wipes the forehead and digital presses Jingming (BL1), separately wipes the Yingxiang (LI20), Shuigou(DU20) and Chengjiang(RN24) for 3 – 5 times respectively,

which is to be repeated 3 times, and then, with the tips of the thumb and fingers, from Shuaigu(GB8) to Naokong(GB19), sweep-disperse the temple for 20 - 30 times, and joins from the temporo-occipital to the neck; after that, grasps with the palmar sides of the fingers along Shaoyang, Taiyang and Du channels in succession for 3 - 5 times.

3) The doctor stands on one side behind the patient and flat-pushes the chest and back, the hypochondriac region, the upper abdomen and the lumbosacral portion for 30 - 50 times.

4) The doctor lifts and grasps two Jianjing(GB21), upper arms and forearm for 35 times; restores the thumbs and four fingers and splits the cracks between fingers for one time respectively; set the shoulders back and forth for 3 circuits respectively; foulaging arms to-and-fro for 3 times; shakes the shoulders and arms 3 - 5 times; pinch-grasps Hegu(LI4) till there is a sensation of aching and distention.

5) Repeat Operation 3.

6) The doctor vibrates fontanel with the center of the palm; and Dazhui (DU14) and the Baliao points(BL31 - 34) with fist back for 3 times respectively.

4. Modification of Manipulation According to Different Syndromes

1) Type of Deficiency of the Liver-Yin and Kidney-Yin: In addition, knead Ganshu(BL18), Shenshu(BL23) and Sanyinjiao(SP6).

2) Type of Insufficiency of both the Spleen and Kidney: In addition, knead Xinshu(BL15), Shenshu(BL23) and Mingmen(DU4).

3) Type of Breakdown of Normal Physiological Coordination between the Heart and the Kidney: in addition, knead Xinshu(BL15) and Shenshu(BL23), and scrub Yongquan(KI1).

4) Type of Deficiency of Qi and Blood in the Heart and Spleen: In addition, knead Xinshu(BL15), Pishu(BL20), Weishu(BL21), Zhongwan(RN12), and Zusanli(ST36).

5) Type of Stagnation of the Liver-qi: In addition, knead Ganshu(BL18), Danshu(BL19), Qimen(LR14) and Yanglingquan(GB34).

5. Course of Treatment: Once a day, 10 times as one course with an interval of 5 - 7 days between two courses.

VI. THERAPEUTIC METHODS
BY CHINESE MEDICATED DIET

1. Dietetic Chinese Drugs

1) Pig brain Fresh pig brain, from whose meninges small blood vessels are removed, is washed clean and used singly to make soup or be braized in brown sauce for eating. It is applicable to the type of syndrome marked by hyperactivity of fire due to yin deficiency with breakdown of the normal physiological coordination between the heart and the kidney.

2) Longan aril (Arillus Longan) Longan aril is taken raw, 12 to 15 g at a time, applicable to the type of syndrome marked by deficiency of qi, blood, heart and spleen. It has a certain curative effect on insomnia and palpitation.

2. Composite Recipes of Chinese Medicated Diet

1) Decoction with Dried Longan Aril and Arborvitae Seeds (Guiyuan Baiziren Tang)

Recipe

Arillus Longan	10 g
Semen Biotae	10 g

Process Put 10 g of dried longan aril and 10 g of arborvitae seeds together into a small aluminium pan, add 500 ml of cold water and half a spoonful of white sugar, cook them together over a slow fire for 20 to 30 minutes until about 200 ml of extract is left, then take the pan away from the fire, remove the residues of the arborvitae seeds and take it as a refreshment. It is applicable to deficiency of qi, blood, heart and spleen.

2) Decoction with Lily Bulb and Arborvitae Seed (Baihe Baiziren Tang)

Recipe

Bulbus Lilii	50 g
Semen Biotae	10 g

Process Put 50 g of fresh lily bulb and 10 g of arborvitae seeds in a small aluminium pan, add 500 ml of cold water and heat it over a slow fire for 20 to 30 minutes. Take it away from the fire, add a spoonful of honey, remove the residues of the arborvitae seeds and eat it as a refreshment.

3) Soft Extract for Calming the Liver, Invigorating the Spleen and Tranquillizing the Mind (Pinggan Yipi Anshen Gao)

Recipe

Arillus Longan	1000 g
Fructus Ziziphi Jujubae	500 g
Spica Prunellae	200 g
Semen Ziziphi Spinosae	100 g
Mel	1000 g
crystal sugar	250 g

Process Put the Chinese-dates, prunella spike and spiny jujube seeds into a big earthenware pot and soak them in cold water for half an hour and then, heat it over a medium fire. When the water boils, decoct it over a slow fire for an hour until 1000 ml or so of extract is left; filter it to get the first extract; add 1500 ml of cold water into the pot and heat it again until 700 ml of medicinal fluid is left; filter it to get the second extract and remove the residues. Put all the extract, the dried longan aril, honey and crystal sugar into the big earthenware pot and heat it over a slow fire for about an hour. Cool it to have soft syrupy extract, and then, put it into a bottle and cover it tight.

Directions Take it after infusion with boiling water, twice a day, 10 to 15 g a time. As for the longan aril, swallow it after chewing it. It is very effective for those who suffer from the flaring of liver-fire marked by irritability accompanied with high blood pressure if they take this kind of soft extract frequently over a long period of time.

Both of the above-mentioned recipes are applicable to the type of syndrome in which liver-fire flares up and burns the heart-yin.

4) Decoction with Dragon's Bone, Oyster Shell and Lotus Seed (Longgu Muli Lianzi Tang)

Recipe

Os Draconis Fossilia Ossis Mastodi	10 g
Concha Ostreae	15 g
Rhizoma Anemarrhenae	3 g
Semen Nelumbinis	30 g

Process Decoct the dragon's bone and oyster shell first, then, put in the rhizome of wind-weed, lotus seeds and white sugar to make decoction for drinking. It exerts a remarkable effect upon those suffering from insomnia, night sweat, dysphoria with smothery sensation and is applicable to the type of hyperactivity of fire due to yin deficiency with breakdown of the normal physiological coordination between the heart and the kidney.

5) Pearl Powder Mixed with Honey (Zhenzhu Mi)

Recipe

Pulvis Margaritae	60 g
Mel	500 g

Process Put 60 g of pearl powder into 500 g of honey and mix them thoroughly, then put it in a bottle.

Directions Take it once a day, 10 g a time, after it is infused with a small quantity of boiling water. Take it for two months as a course of treatment.

6) Honey with Sesame Seed and Three Kinds of Kernels (San Ren Zhima Mi)

Recipe

Semen Ziziphi Spinosae	60 g
Semen Biotae	60 g
Fructus Cannabis	30 g
Semen Sesami Nigrum	500 g
Mel	500 g

Process First, decoct the arborvitae seeds, hemp seeds and spiny jujube seeds; put the first and the second extract obtained separately and honey into an earthenware pot to be heated over a small fire. When it boils, put in the roasted black sesame seeds, stir it continuously with a chopstick for a quarter of an hour, then, remove the pot from the fire: Put the content into a bottle after it cools.

Directions Take it twice a day, 10 g at a time, after infusing it with boiling water or take it with cooked rice (or millet) water. As for the sesame seeds, swallow it after it chewing. This recipe is especially fit for the aged patients who suffer from neurosis.

Chapter Four
Cerebrovascular Accidents

Cerebrovascular accident, or stroke, is a focal neurologic disorder due to a pathologic process in a blood vessel. In most cases the onset is abrupt and evolution rapid, and symptoms reach a peak within seconds, minutes or hours. Partial or complete recovery may occur over a period of hours to months.

Occlusion of a cerebral artery by thrombosis or embolism results in a cerebral infarction with its associated clinical effects. Other conditions may on occasion also produce cerebral infarction and thus may be confused with cerebral arteritis, systemic hypotension, reactions to cerebral angiography, and transient cerebral ischemia.

Cerebral hemorrhage is usually caused by rupture of an arteriosclerotic cerebral vessel. Subarachnoid hemorrhage is usually due to rupture of a congenitally weak blood vessel or aneurysm.

Transient cerebral ischemia may also occur without producing a cerebral infarction. Premonitory recurrent focal cerebral ischemic attacks may occur and are apt to be in a repetitive pattern in a given case. Attack may last for 10 seconds to one hour, but the average duration is 2 to 10 minutes. As many as several hundred such attacks may occur. In some instances of transient ischemia, the neurologic deficit may last up to 20 hours.

Narrowing of the extracranial arteries (particularly the internal carotid artery at its origin in the neck and, in some cases, the intrathoracic arteries) by arteriosclerotic patches has been incriminated in a significant number of cases of transient cerebral ischemias and infarction.

In traditional Chinese medicine, the disease is considered to be caused by stirring wind arising from hyperactivity of Yang in the liver which results from exasperation or agitation accompanied with disturbance of the Zang-fu organs. Qi and blood imbalance of Yin and Yang and dysfunction of the channels and collaterals. Another factor is endogenous wind caused by phlegm- heat after over-indulgence in alcohol and fatty diet.

I. CLINICAL MANIFESTATIONS

Early phase. Variable degrees and types occur. The onset may be violent, with the patient falling to the ground and lying like a person in deep sleep, with flushed, face, stertorous or cheyne-stroke respirations, full and slow pulse, and one arm and leg usually flaccid. Death may occur in a few hours or days. Lesser grades of stroke may consist of slight derangement of speech, thought, motion, sensation, or vision. Consciousness need not be altered. Symptoms may last seconds to minutes or longer or may persist unremittingly for an indefinite period. Some degree of recovery is usual.

Premonitory symptoms may include headache, dizziness, drowsiness, and mental confusion. Focal premonitory symptoms are more likely to occur with thrombosis.

Generalized neurologic signs are most common with cerebral hemorrhage and include fever, headache, vomiting, convulsion, and coma. Nuchal rigidity is frequent with subarachnoid hemorrhage or intracerebral hemorrhage. Mental changes are commonly noted in the period following a stroke and may include confusion, disorientation and memory defects.

II. MAIN POINTS OF DIAGNOSIS

1. Sudden onset of neurologic complaints varying from focal motor or hypesthesia and speech defects to profound coma.

2. May be associated with vomiting, convulsions or headaches.

3. Nuchal rigidity frequently found.

III. TREATMENT OF COMMON SYNDROMES

1. When the patient complains of disorientation, coughing with rales, coma, chest distress, with whitish glossy coating of the tongue and slippery pulse, the following formula is given.

Dao Tan Tang Jia Jian

Recipe

Dried old orange peel	12 g
Pinellia	10 g
Tuckahoe	10 g
Licorice root	6 g
Jack-in-the-pulpit	10 g
Fruit of immature crtron or trifoliate orange	10 g
Bulb of fritillary	10 g
Tabasheer	10 g
Root of purple-flowered peucedanum	15 g
Apricot kernel	12 g
Root of the narrow-leaved polygala	12 g
Grass-leaved sweetflag	12 g

Decoction and Dosage   All the above herbs make a dose and six to ten doses are prescribed with one dose daily. Each dose is simmered twice and then the broth of each mixed, half of the mixed broth each time, twice a day.

2. When the patient has muscular atrophy and debility of the lower limbs with impaired mobility of the knees and ankle joints, which are caused by empty blood vessels, malnutrition of the muscles of the lower limbs, sensory disturbance of the skin, the following formula is prescribed.

Bu Yang Huan Wu Tang (Decoction for invigorating yang)

Recipe

Milk veteh	40 g
Chinese angelica	30 g
Unpeeled root of herbaceous peony	30 g
Szechwan lovage rhizome	20 g
Earthworm	15 g
Peach kernel	12 g
Safflower	12 g
Cassia	12 g
Achyranthes root	15 g
Scorpion	10 pieces
Root of red rooted salcia	30 g
Liquorice	6 g

The decoction and dosage the same as that of Dao Tan Tang.

In addition, infections prepared from the root of red rooted salvia and Szechwan lovage rhizome are also very effective. 40 ml of red rooted salvia injection and 250 to 500 ml of 10% glucose can be given intravenously once daily and a course lasts two weeks. Injection of Szechwan lovage rhizome can be given alone intramuscularly, 80 mg each time, or together with 500 ml of 4% glucose once daily intravenously.

IV. ACUPUNCTURE THERAPY

Acupuncture therapy is indispensable at the stage of recovery and convalescence.

There two types of windstroke according to the degree of severity: the severe type and the mild type.

1. The Severe Type   In this type, the Zang-fu organs are attacked and the symptoms are manifested in the channels, collaterals and the viscerae. The severe type can further be divided into two subtypes:

A. The Tense Syndrome   The chief manifestations of this type are sudden collapse, coma, staring eyes, clenched fists and jaws, redness of face and ears, gurgling with sputum, coarse breathing, retention of urine, and constipation, wiry and rolling forceful pulse. The prescription for puncture is as follows:

Main points: Shuigou(DU26), Baihui(DU20), Yongquan(KI1).

Auxiliary points: Jiache(ST6), Xiaguan(ST7) and Hegu(LI4) for clenched jaws; Tiantu(RN22) and Fenglong(ST40) for gurgling with sputum; Yamen (DU15), Lieque(LI7) and Tongli(HT5) for aphasia and stiffness of the tongue.

Method: All the main points are prescribed with the corresponding auxiliary points according to the symptoms and the puncture is moderate. The needle are retained for 15 minutes and the treatment is given once daily.

B. The flaccid syndrome   The chief manifestations of this type are coma, ralxed hands, agape mouth, closed eyes, pallor, profuse drops of sweat over head and face, and snoring. There may also be incontinence of feces and urine, cold limbs and feeble pulse. The prescription for puncture is:

Points: Quchi(LI11), Guanyuan(RN4) and Shenque(RN8).

Method: All the above points are punctured with moderate stimulation. The needles are retained for 20 minutes and the therapy is given once daily.

2. The Mild Type   In this type, only the channels and collaterals are attacked and the symptoms pertain only to the channels and collaterals. The symptoms and signs are mostly those of the sequelae of the severe type, which involve the channels and collaterals. There are also primary cases without affliction of Zang-fu organs. Manifestations are hemiplegia or deviation of mouth due to motor or sensory impairment.

For hemiplegia: This may be severe or mild and the attack may be on either side of the body. At the beginning, the affected limbs may be limbs and later they become stiff, which finally leads to motor impairment. There may be dizziness and dysphasia.

Main points: Baihui(DU20), Fengfu(DU16) and Tongtian(BL7).

Auxiliary points: Jianyu(LI15), Quchi(LI11), Waiguan(SJ5) and Hegu (LI4) for upper extremities; Huantiao(GB30), Yanglingquan(GB24) and Zusanli(ST36) for lower extremities.

Method: All the main points are prescribed with the corresponding auxiliary points according to the symptoms. The needles are retained for 20 minutes and the therapy is given once daily.

V. PROPHYLACTIC MEASURES

Senile patients with deficiency of Qi and excessive sputum or with manifestations of hyperactivity of liver yang such as dizziness and palpitation may sometimes present symptoms of stiffness of tongue, slurred speech and numbness of finger tips. There are prodromal signs of windstroke. Prophylactic measures are emphasizing diet and daily activities, avoiding over- straining. Frequent moxibustion on Zusanli(ST36) and Xuanzhong(BL39) may prevent the attacks.

Chapter Five
Cerebrovascular Accidental Sequela

The disease refers to hemiplegia, slurred speech, deviation of the mouth and eye, and others caused by acute cerebrovascular diseases, pertaining to the category of "wind stroke" in traditional Chinese medicine.

I. MAIN SYMPTOMS AND SIGNS

Hemiplegia, numbness of the muscles and skin, deviation of the mouth and eye, slurred speech or aphasia, numbness, atrophy, weakness and apraxia of the hand and foot, etc..

II. TREATMENT BY ACUPUNCTURE

1. Body Acupuncture

Prescription: Baihui(DU20), Fengchi(DU16) and Tianchuang(SI16).

Supplemtary Points: For paralysis of the upper limbs, Jianyu(LI15), Quchi(LI11), Waiguan(SJ5) and Hegu(LI4) are added; for paralysis of the lower limbs, Huantiao(GB30), Yanglingquan(GB34), Zusanli(ST36) and Juegu(GB39); for deviation of the mouth and eye, Dicang(ST4) and Jiache (ST6).

Method: Use the filiform needles to puncture the points with the even movement method, or puncture the points alternatively, first those on the healthy side and then those on the affected side.

2. Scalp Acupunture

Prescription: Contralateral motor area, sensory area, foot motor sensory area, speech areas.

Method: Use filiform needles to puncture the areas along the skin. Twirl the needles at intervals. Retain them for 30 minutes or electrify them for 50 minutes. It is better for the patient to feel warm, numb, distending and subsultory on the affected limb.

III. THERAPEUTIC METHODS
BY PRACTISING QIGONG

1. Self-Treatment by Practising Qigong

1) Basic Maneuvers

It is advisable to practise Upper Limbs Qigong and Lower Limbs Qigong.

2) Auxiliary Maneuvers

Those suffering from facial paralysis are advised to practise Head and Face Qigong.

2. External Qi Maneuvers

1) Basic Maneuvers

(1) Press, knead and pinch Hegu(LI4), Jiache(ST6), Neiguan(PC6), Quchi(LI11), Yanglingquan(GB34), Weizhong(BL40) and the bilateral sides of the fingernails.

(2) First knead the region where Urinary Bladder Meridian distributes on the back from above to below 6-7 times.

(3) Apply the flat-palm form or the sword-fingers form, use the pushing, pulling and leading manipulations to emit qi onto Yintang(EX-HN3) and Baihui (DU20), then conduct qi along the Ren Channel to flow down to Guanyuan (RN4). Then apply the same method to conduct the channel qi downward along the Urinary Bladder Meridian and the Stomach Meridian so as to make qi sensation balanced from above to below and from left to right.

2) Auxiliary Maneuvers

(1) Right hemiplegia: First tip and knead the right Hanyan(GB4) and Jiao-

sun(SJ20), sweep the cephalic region where the Gall Bladder Meridian passes, then employ the flat-palm form, the pulling and leading manipulations to emit qi onto the left side of the head and conduct qi to flow down to the neck and cross to the right Stomach Meridian and the Urinary Bladder Meridian to flow down to the feet.

(2) Left hemiplegia: Employ the above method to conduct qi from the right to the left side.

IV. COMPOSITE RECIPES OF
CHINESE MEDICATED DIET

1. Gruel of Bamboo Juice (Zhuli Zhou)
Recipe
Succus Bambosae
Semen Setariae Italicae
Process
Get henon bamboo juice (excreted from the baked bamboo stem) and millet, each equal in portion; first, make gruel with the millet, and when it is done, put in the bamboo juice. Stir and mix it thoroughly for eating.

2. Drink of Waxgourd Seeds (Dongguazi Yin)
Recipe
Semen Benincasae   30 g
brown sugar right amount
Process
Mash 30 g of waxgourd seeds and an appropriate amount of brown sugar; taek it after infusing it with boiling water.

3. Gruel of Bush-cherry Seed (Yuliren Zhou)
Recipe
Semen Pruni   10 g
Semen Oryzae Sativae   60 g
Process

Grind 10 g of bush-cherry seeds with 100 ml of water, and filter it to get the extract; then, add water until the mixture amounts to 1000 ml. Put in 60 g of polished round-grained rice to make gruel for eating.

The three recipes listed above are applicable to the type of phlegm and heat accumulated in the interior.

4. Tea with Sword-bean Root (Daodou Cha)

    Recipe

Radix Canavaliae	30 g
ric ewine or black tea	3 g

Process

Decoct 30 g of sword-bean root with 3 g of rice (or millet) wine or black tea to make a drink for oral administration.

5. Gruel with Fresh-water Mussel (Bang Zhou)

    Recipe

Concha Margaritifera Usta	120 g
Semen Oryzae Sativae	50 g

Process

Make gruel for eating with 120 g of fresh-water mussel and 50 g of polished round-grained rice.

6. Powder of Pig's Bile and Green Gram (Zhudan Ludou Fen)

    Recipe

Succus Fellis Suillum	120 g
Semen Phaseoli Radiati	80 g

Process

Mix 80 g of green gram flour thoroughly with 120 g of pig's bile and dry it by airing, then, grind it into fine powder. Take 6 g twice daily.

The three recipes listed above have a certain curative effect on the type of blazing of liver-fire.

7. Ginseng Decoction (Renshen Tang)

    Recipe

Radix Ginseng	10 g
Pericarpium Citri Reticulatae	10 g
Folium Perillae	15 g

granulated sugar	150 g

Process

Decoct 10 g of ginseng, 10 g of tanerine peel, 15 g of purple perilla leaves and 150 g of granulated sugar in 3000 ml of water. Take it as a drink.

8. Decoction of Schisandra Fruit (Wuweizi Tang)

Recipe	
Fructus Schisandrae	10 g
Folium Perillae	18 g
Radix Ginseng	12 g
granulated sugar	100 g

Process

Get 10 g of schisandra fruit, 18 g of purple perilla leaves, 12 g of ginseng and 100 g of granulated sugar. Decoct the first three drugs in 3000 ml of water until 1500 ml is left; remove the dregs and let it settle; and add in the granulated sugar. It can be taken as much as one likes.

9. Powder of Oyster Shell and Wheat Bran (Muli Maifu San)

Recipe

Concha Ostreae

Exocarpium Fructi Tritici

Process

Have oyster shell powder and wheat bran mixed thoroughly, each equal in portion. Take 3 g at a time, twice a day.

The three recipes mentioned above have a good preventive effect on the syndrome of feeble vital-qi tending to break, so patients who suffer from this syndrome may choose one or two from them for use.

10. Drink of Wolfberry Fruit and Ophiopogon Root (Gou Mai Yin)

Recipe

Fructus Lycii

Radix Ophiopogonis

Process

Decoct wolfberry fruit and ophiopogon roots each equal in portion. It can be taken as a drink.

11. Gruel of Rehmannia Root (Dihuang Zhou)

Recipe

Succus Radicis Rehmanniae   100 ml

Semen Oryzae Sativae

Process

Get 100 ml of the juice of rehmannia roots ready for use; first, make gruel with polished round-grained rice and when it is done, put in the juice of rehmannia root and stir thoroughly before eating.

12. Gruel of Lucid Asparagus Root (Tianmendong Zhou)

Recipe

Radix Asparagi   30 g

Semen Oryzae Sativae   50 g

Process

Make gruel for eating with 30 g of lucid asparagus root and 50 g of polished round-grained rice.

13. Gruel of Chinese Yam and Yolk (Shuyu Jizihuang Zhou)

Recipe

yolks of cooked eggs 3

Rhizoma Dioscoreae

Process

Put three yolks of cooked eggs into gruel of Chinese yam for use.

The above four recipes are applicable to the type of deficiency of the kidney and blockade of the channels and collaterals.

Chapter Six
Viral Encephalitis

Encephalitis may be defined as an inflammatory process of the CNS that results in altered function of various portions of the brain and spinal cord and is usually accompanied by signs of systemic infection.

Viral encephalitis may be characterized by: 1. A mild abortive infection; 2. A type of illness clinically indistinguishable from aseptic meningitis; and 3. A severe involvement of the CNS. The latter is often characterized by a sudden onset, high fever, meningeal signs, stupor, disorientation, tremors, convulsions, spasticity, coma and death. Case fatality ranges from 1% to 34.9%. The sequelae are more common in infants. A specific diagnosis can be made either by demonstrating a rise in the level of antibody in the serum of the convalescent patient or by isolating a virus from the CNS or CSF.

In traditional Chinese medicine, the condition is considered to be caused by epidemic Qi, a pathogenic factor of high infectivity. The terms of diagnosis are "acute or fulminating infectious disease in summer." or "summer-heat convulsion." or "acute febrile with prolonged onset."

I. CLINICAL MANIFESTATIONS

There are many types of viral encephalitides. They vary from benign forms, resembling aseptic meningitis, lasting a few days and are followed by complete recovery to fulminating encephalitis with the clinical manifestations of paresis, sensory changes, convulsions, increased intracranial pressure, coma and death.

The onset of viral encephalitis may be sudden or gradual and is marked by fever, headache, dizziness, vomiting, apathy and stiffenss of the neck. Ataxia, tremors, mental confusion, speech difficulties, stupor or hyperexcitability, delirium, convulsions and coma, and death may follow. In some cases there may be a prodromal period of 1 to 4 days characterized by chills and fever, headache, malaise, sore throat, conjunctivitis, and pains in the extremities and abdomen followed by encephalitic signs just mentioned. Abortive forms with headache and fever only or a syndrome resembling aseptic meningitis may occur.

The variations in the clinical patterns of encephalitis depend on the distribution, location and concentration of neuronal lesions. Ocular palsies and ptosis are uncommon. Cerebellar incoordination is seen. Flaccid paralysis of the extremities resembling that of poliomyelitis is sometimes encountered. Paralysis of the shoulder girdle muscle is described as a singular feature of a tick-bonee encephalitis.

The CSF is clear and manometric readings of pressure vary from normal to markedly elevated. As a rule, pleocytosis of 40 to 400 cells, chiefly mononuclear, is found. The protein and glucose values may be slightly elevated or normal.

II. MAIN POINTS OF DIAGNOSIS

A diagnosis of acute encephalitis is indicated by the clinical findings. The circumstances in which the disease occurs are important. The specific type of encephalitis can be determined only by isolation and identification of the virus or by demonstration of the formation of or rise of level of antibody in convalescence. Arboviruses are rarely detected in the CSF, blood or other material during life. It is generally fruitless and inappropriate to search for them except in CNS tissue removed with sterile precautions at necropsy. A serologic diagnosis may be reached by means of complement fixation or hemagglutination- inhibition test. Paired serum specimens are necessary. The first should be drawn as soon after onset as possible and the second, 2 or 3 weeks later.

III. DIFFERENTIATION AND TREATMENT OF COMMON SYNDROMES

1. Acute Febrile Disease with Prolonged Onset

Acute febrile disease with rather prolonged latencies after the pathogenic warm factor entering the body any time in the four seasons is characterized by the symptoms complex of internal heat at the onset. The chief symptoms are fever, ehadache, perspiration, chilly sensation, pain in the throat, thirst, stiffness of the neck, mental confusion, delirium, convulsions, thin white or slight yellowish coating of the tongue and rapid pulse. The principle for treatment is to purify the Qi with pungent-cold drugs and to detoxify the body. The formula of first choice is Bai Hu Tang Jia Jian.

Recipe

Gypsum	60 g
Root of Zhejiang figwort	30 g
Tuber of dwarf lilyturf	30 g
Fresh or dried rehmannia	30 g
Rhizome of wind-weed	12 g
Honeysuckle flower	30 g
Weeping forsythia fruit	30 g
Common red rhizome	30 g
Dryers woad root	30 g
Dryers woad leaf	30 g
Cicada slough	20 g
Larva of a silkworm with batrytis	10 g
Licorie root	6 g

Decoction and Dosage

All the above herbs make a dose and six to ten doses are prescribed with one dose daily. Each dose is simmered twice and then the broth of each mixed, half of the mixed broth each time, twice a day.

2. Acute Febrile Disease with the Invasion of the Heat into the Pericardium

The onset of this type is either sudden or gradual and marked by fever, headache, mental confusion, stupor, delirium, tremors, yellow coating of the tongue with dark red color, and full pulse. the treatment is to purge the pathogenic fire and calm the wind with Qi Ying Tang Jia Jian.

Recipe

Gypsum	60 g
Rhizome of wind-weed	12 g
Fresh or dried rehmannia	20 g
Root of Zhejiang figwort	30 g
Root-bark of peony	15 g
Dyers woad root	30 g
Dyers woad leaf	30 g
Rhubarb	10 g
Jack-in-the-pulpit	12 g
Tabasheer	12 g
Earthworm	15 g
Scorpion	7-15 pieces
Centipede	1 or 2 pieces
Buffalo horn	30 g

3. Acute Febrile Disease due to Disturbance of the Heart by Phlegmatic Fire

Thermal pathogen in combination with "phlegm" causes mental disturbances. The main symptoms are mental confusion, delirium, mania and excitability, or spitting sputum and saliva, red tongue with yellowish and glossy coating, slippery and rapid pulse. The treatment is to reduce phlegm for resuscitation with Dao Tan Tang Jia Jian.

Recipe

Dried old orange peel	12 g
Pinellia	12 g

Tuckahoe	10 g
Licorice root	6 g
Jack-in-the-pulpit	12 g
Fruit of immature citron or trifoliate orange	12 g
Tabasheer	12 g
Grass-leaved sweetflag	12 g
Root-tuber of aromatic turmeric	12 g
Bamboo Shavings	12 g
Musk	0.06 g
Bamboo juice	3 or 4 spoonful

4. Acute Febrile Disease Caused by Inward Invasion of the Weak Wind

Diseases due to impariment of Yin and deficiency of blood mainfest poor maintenance of msucles and tendons, and produce symptoms simulating the wind movements such as dizziness, convulsions or tremor, flushed face, hot palms and soles, dysphoria, restlessness, insomnia, dry throat and mouth, dark red tongue with reduced saliva, weak and rapid pulse. The treatment is to calm the "wind" by nourishing the Yin. The commonly used formula is Da Ding Feng Zhu Jia Jian.

Recipe	
Root of herbaceous	30 g
Donkey-hide gelatin	12 g
Tortoise plastron	20 g
Dried rehmannia	20 g
Fructus cannabis	20 g
Hemp seed	20 g
Fruit of Chinese magnaliavine	20 g
Tuber of dwarf lilyturf	30 g
Oyster	30 g
Turtle-shell	30 g
Licorice root	6 g
Egg core	6 g

Certain ready-made herb pills such as An Gong Niu Huang Pill, Niu Huang Qing Xin Pill, Zi Xue Dan and Zhi Bao Dan are also very effective for the conditions.

IV. ACUPUNCTURE THERAPY

1. For Paralysis of the Upper Limbs

Points: Jianyu(LI15), Quchi(LI11), Hegu(LI4) and Waiguan(SJ5).

2. For Paralysis of the Lower Limbs

Points: Biguan(ST31), Zusanli(ST36), Jiexi(ST41), Huantiao(GB30), Yanglingquan(GB34) and Xuanzhong(GB39).

3. For Convulsion

Points: Zhongwan(RN12), Guanyuan(RN4), Zusanli(ST36), Zhangmen (LR13), Yintang(EX-HN3).

4. For Eye Deviation

Points: Hegu (LI4), Jingming (BL1), Fengchi (GB20), Taiyang (EX-HN5), Xingjian(LR2).

Method: All the points are punctured with moderate stimulation and the needles are retained for 20 minutes. The therapy is given once daily.

Chapter Seven
Toxic Encephalopathy

Toxic encephalopathy, characterized by hyperspasmia and disturbance of consciousness, blongs to "infantile convulsion" in traditional Chinese medicine. In acute stage, it belongs to acute infantile convulsion, manifested by sudden onset, quick progress and high fever. In recovery stage, it belongs to slow infantile convulsion, marked by weakened pathogenic heat and damaged yin-type body fluid. The symptoms of toxic encephalopathy are similar to those of encephalitis, mostly occur in the toxic progress of infectious diseases, such as pneumonia, bacillary dysentery, whooping cough and upper respiratory tract infection. It is usually considered as an allergy of human body to the toxin, due to edema degeneration caused by lacking oxygen in brain cells, not due to invasion of pathogens directly to the central nervous system. It usually occur in the children between two and ten years old.

I. ETIOLOGY AND PATHOGENESIS

Young children usually has more yang and less yin. The pathogens, after invading the child, usually change into heat. Excess heat will stir up liver-wind and fire the body fluid into phlegm which may stuff up the clear orifices. Therefore, the pahtogenesis in the acute stage may be summarized as heat, phlegm, wind and convulsion. The pathological changes develop mainly in the heart and liver. In recovery stage, it is mostly caused by damaged yin due to febrile diseases, insufficiency of kidney-yin, unmoistened liver, and stirred wind due to deficient yin, or by damaged spleen and stomach. In short, the disease of this stage is related to the spleen, liver and kidney.

1. Invasion of Seasonal Pathogens

It may be caused by pathogens such as wind, coldness, summer-heat, dryness and fire, especially by the affection of wind pathogen in winter and spring, summer-heat pathogen in summer and autumn, and seasonal infectious pathogens.

(1) Invasion of Wind Pathogen

Wind pathogen, main etiology for every disease, usually invades people together with cold and heat. Because of lack of yin and surplus of yang in young children, the invaded pathogens are easily transformed into heat and the excess heat into fire, then stir up wind. Wind and fire stir up each other, leading to convulsion. If the pathogenic heat fires the body fluid into phlegm, the orifices will be stuffed up with presenting unconsciousness. If the air passage is obstructed, short breath and flaring of nares will be seen. If the heat changes into fire and attacks Jueyin inwards, coma and convulsion will occur.

(2) Invasion of Summer Pathogen

The solid and hollow organs of young children are tender and weak, the vital yin energy is not enough. They are apt to be affected by summer-heat in very hot weather which belongs to pathogenic yang and can change into fire most quickly. When the pathogenic heat and fire invade Jueyin Meridians, attack pericardium adversely, coma and convulsion will be seen.

(3) Invasion of Epidemic Pathogens

If the young children with latent phlegm in the interior are attacked by epidemic pathogens, the pathogen wrestle with each other, firing the body fluid into phlegm, obstructing the air passage. As a result, the pathogenic heat stagnates in the interior and goes up to stuff the clear orifices, thus developing coma and convulsion.

2. Damp-heat Epidemic Pathogens

When food taken is unclean, the damp-heat epidemic pahtogens enter the body through mouth, stagnate in the stomach and intestines and change rapidly into fire and invade inwards Jueyin Meridians, developing coma and convulsion. If the body resistance is vigorous while the pathogens are sthenia, there will occur the excess sysndrome of stroke and heat, marked by sudden onset and persistent high fever, and frequent convulsion. If the pathogens are violently exuberant, the vital-qi has been damaged interiorly and fails to prevail over pathogens, the excess syndrome of stroke will be seen clinically. It is probably combined with the external prostration syndrome due to exhausted yang. There occurs a complex situation of unconsciousness and collapse, and of co- existence of cold and heat. Stagnation of qi and blood due to accumulation of pathogens in the interior will develop. Such symptoms will occur as abdominal pain and tenesmus for stagnation of qi, pus blood due to blood stasis.

II. MAIN POINTS OF DIAGNOSIS

1. This disease may occur at any age, but usually infants from 1 to 3 years old. The symptoms of brain damage often follow the primary disorders within a few days or 1-2 weeks after their attack.

2. The clinical manifestations are various. The onset is usually abrupt with high fever, headache, vomiting, restlessness or lethargy, convulsion, coma, bulging of anterior fontanelle, platycoria, and delayed reaction to light, often accompanied with holotonia, decerebrate rigidity or opisthotonos, and unilateral or bilateral paralysis. Some patients may have the symptoms of meningeal irritation, increased or reduced tendon reflex, and also have cerebellar symptoms, such as ataxia, nystagmus and kinetic tremor.

3. Laboratory examinations show that cerebrospinal fluid is clear. All are normal except that the pressure is high and sometimes there is a slight increase of protein in cerebrospinal fluid.

4. Arteriolar spasm, blood stasis of the small vein and retinal edema or papilledema can be observed by fundus examination.

III. DIFFERENTIATION AND
TREATMENT OF COMMON SYNDROMES

The primary disease should be treated before starting the treatment of the disease.

1. Invasion of Exogenous Wind Pathogens (Often seen at the early stage of

the complicated toxic encephalopathy secondary to the upper respiratory tract infection or pneumonia).

Main Symptoms and Signs: Fever, headache, cough and running nose, sore throat, irritability or flaring of nares, sudden coma and convulsion, red tongue with yellow fur.

Therapeutic Method: Dispelling wind and heat to relieve the stagnated lung; inducing rsuscitation and relieving convulsion.

Recipe: Yinqiao San(Powder of Lonicera and Forsythia) and Ma Xing Shi Gan Tang (Decoction of Ephedra, Apricot Kernel, Gypsum and Liquorice), modified.

Flos Lonicerae	15 g
Herba Ephedrae Praeparatae	6 g
Semen Armeniacae Amarum Praeparatae	3 g
Gypsum Fibrosum	24 g
Fructus Forsythiae	9 g
Flos Chrysanthemi	9 g
Ramulus Uncariae cum Uncis	9 g
Rhizoma Acori Graminei	9 g
Fructus Arctii	9 g
Bombyx Batryticatus	6 g
Caulis Bambusae in Taeniam	6 g
Radix Glycyrrhizae	3 g

Decoct the above drugs for oral use.

Modification: In case of severe cold-syndrome of superficies, marked by stuffing nose and obvious flaring of nares, Herba Ephedrae 6 g should be used instead of Herba Ephedrae Praeparatae, and additional Herba Asari 3 g should be used to promote the power of dispelling the pathogens from superificies. In case of dyspepsia, fullness of the abdomen and thick greasy fur on the tongue, Fructus Cnataegi Praeparatae 12 g, Semen Arecae 12 g should be added to promote digestion and remove stagnated food. If the disease complicates whooping cough, Spica Prunellae 15 g, Lumbricus 9 g, Fructus Aurantii Immaturus 6 g, Radix Asteris 9 g and Fructus Trichosanthis 15 g should be added to relieve cough and resolve phlegm. If the disease occurs in hot summer, modified Xiangru Yin (Decoction of Herba Elsholtziae seu Moslae) should be used instead.

2. Invasion of Damp-heat Epidemic Pathogens (Often seen at the early stage of toxic encephalopathy secondary to bacillary dysentery).

Main Symptoms and Signs: Sudden onset, persistent high fever, irritability and reslessness, thirst with desire of drinking, coma and delirium, frequent convulsion, probably followed by glutinous stinking stools with pus blood, crimson tongue with yelowish dry fur.

Therapeutic Method: Removing heat and dampness; calming the endopathic wind to induce resuscitation.

Recipe: Gegen Qinlian Tang (Decoction of Radix Puerariae, Radix Scutellariae and Rhizoma Coptidis) and Baitouwong Tang, modified.

Radix Pueraria	12 g
Radix Scutellariae	12 g
Cortex Fraxini	9 g
Rhizoma Coptidis	6 g
Herba Portulacae	15 g
Fructus Crataegi Praeparata	12 g
Semen Arecae	12 g
Ramulus Uncariae cum Uncis	9 g
Rhizoma Acori Graminei	9 g
Radix Curcumae	9 g
Scorpio	6 g

Decoct the above drugs for oral use.

Modification: In case of productive sputum and saliva with pharyngeal rale, Succus Bambosae 10 ml and Arisaema cum Bile 6 g should be added to remove phlegm and to cause resuscitation.

3. Intense Heat in Both Qi and Ying Systems

Main Symptoms and Signs: Often seen in the stage of cerebral edema of toxic encephalopathy, in the course of the primary disease, with sudden high fever, headache, vomiting, restlessness, delirium, drowsiness, convulsions of the limbs, stiffness of the extremities and neck, involuntary staring, lockjaw, and unconsciousness, deep-red tongue with yellow and dry fur, either taut and rapid or slippery and rapid pulse.

Therapeutic Principle: Clearing away pathogenic heat from qi and ying systems, arresting convulsions and inducing resuscitation.

Recipe: Modified Antipyretic and Antitoxic Decoction.

Flos Lonicerae	18 g
Fructus Forsythiae	9 g
Radix Coptidis	6 g
Gypsum Fibrosum	30 g
Rhizoma Anemarrhenae	9 g
Cortex Moutan Radicis	9 g
Radix Curcumae	9 g
Rhizoma Acori Graminei	9 g
Cornu Rhinocerotis (Ground into fine powder to be taken after being infused in the finished decoction)	3 g
Pulvis Cornu Saigae (infused)	3 g
Plumula Nelumbinis	3 g

All the above drugs are to be decocted in water for oral administration.

Drugs of cool or cold nature should be used very cautiously when there is pathogenic dampness with thick and greasy tongue coating. Instead, the following drugs should be added: Herba Agastachis 9 g, Herba Eupatorii 9 g, Semen Coicis 15 g, Semen Amomi Cardamomi 6 g.

4. Deficiency of Both Qi and Yin

Main Symptoms and Signs: Often seen in the late stage of toxic encephalopathy with residual low fever, pale and occasional flush of zygomatico-facial region, vexation and insomnia, sluggish look, occasional convulsion, rigidity and paralysis of limbs or dysphagia, blindness, deafness, aphasia, emaciation, spontaneous perspiration, night sweat, deep-red tongue with thin white fur or without fur, thready, weak and rapid pulse.

Recipe: Modified Great Pearl for Wind Syndrome.

Radix Rehmanniae	9 g
Radix Rehmanniae Praeparata	9 g
Radix Paeoniae Alba	12 g
Radix Codonopsis Pilosulae	9 g
Radix Ophiopogonis	12 g

Rhizoma Atractylodis Macrocephlae	9 g
Radix Angelicae Sinensis	9 g
Plastrum Testudinis	9 g
Carapax Trionycis	15 g
Radix Astragali seu Hedysari	15 g
Rhizoma Acori Graminei	9 g

All the above drugs are to be decocted inwater for oral administration.

5. Deficiency of Liver and Kidney

Main Symptoms and Signs: Often seen in the convalescence of toxic encephalopathy with rigidity and spasm of limbs and occasional convulsions or mental disturbance, aphasia or slurred speech, blindness, deafness, red tongue with little fur, and feeble and rapid pulse.

Therapeutic Principle: Nourishing the liver and kidney; promoting blood circulation, dredging the channels and collaterals, and removing phlegm and inducing resuscitation.

Recipe: Modified Prescription of Duqi Pill of Seven Ingredients and Decoction Invigorating Yang for Recuperation.

Radix Rehmanniae Praeparata	9 g
Fructus Corni	9 g
Fructus Lycii	9 g
Radix Angelicae Sinensis	9 g
Poria	12 g
Lumbricus	6 g
Rhizoma Acori Graminei	9 g
Rhizoma Ligustici Chuanxiong	6 g
Flos Carthami	6 g

All the above drugs are to decocted in water for oral adminsitration.

In case of rigidity and spastic of limbs, add 9 grams of Zaocys, 9 grams of Bambyx Batryticatus and 6 grams of Scorpio; for those with flaccid paralysis of limbs and emaciation, add 18 grams Radix Astragali seu Hedysari, 9 grams of Rhizoma Atracty lodis Macrocephalae and 9 grams of Fructus Chaenomelis; for those with blindness and deafness, 9 grams of Fructus Ligustri Lucidi, 9 grams of Herba Dendrobii and 9 grams of Fructus Liquidambaris should be used; and for those with intellectual disturbance, add 12 grams of Fructus Alpiniae Oxyphyllae, 15 grams of Semen Ziziphi Apinosae and 9 grams of Radix Polygalae.

6. Stagnation of Phlegm in Collaterals (Seen in the later period of the recovery stage of the toxic encephalopathy)

Main Symptoms and Signs: Dull appearance, or dementia, aphasia and deafness, irritability, hyperspasmia or stiffness of the trunk and limbs, unstable standing and walking, thin and white greasy fur.

Therapeutic Method: Expelling wind pathogens and disolving phlegm; promoting blood circulation to remove obstruction in the channels and to induce resuscitation.

Recipe: Qianzheng San (Powder for Treating Wry-Mouth) and Wendan Tang (Decoction for Clearing Away Gallbladder-heat), modified.

Rhizoma Typhonii	9 g
Pericarpium Citri Reticulatae	9 g
Bombyx Batryticatus	6 g
Scorpio	6 g
Rhizoma Pinelliae	6 g
Arisaema cum Bile	6 g
Fructus Aurantii Immaturus	6 g
Os Costaziae	12 g
Radix Curcumae	9 g
Rhizoma Acori Graminei	9 g

OTHER THERAPIES

1. Acupuncture Therapy

Acupuncture produces a temporary effect on inducing consciousness and stopping spasm. In case of convulsion, Shuigou (DU26), Hegu (LI4), Neiguan (PC6), Taichong (LR3), Yongquan (KI1), Baihui (DU20) and Yintang (EX-HN3) should be chosen. In case of high fever, Quchi (LI11), Dazhui (DU14) and Shixuan (EX0-UE11) should be chosen. Add Fenglong (ST40) for rale; Xiaguan(ST7) and Jiache(ST6) for trismus. Strong or medium stimulation may be given in every case.

2. External Treatment

Rub their teeth with a black berry when the children suffer from trismus. Chubi San or Tongguan San may be blown into the nose to cause sneeze in order to stop convulsion and induce resuscitation.

PREVENTION AND NURSING

1. Improve constitution to avoid being attacked by external pathogens. Take clean food and drink, keep the surronding sanitation to void invasion of damp-heat pathogens.

2. Cure primary diseases promptly, such as upper respiratory tract infection, pneumonia, bacillary dysentery.

3. Stop spasm and be ready to draw out sputum, saliva, guttural secretions to avoid suffocation.

4. Keep the sick child lying on his back, turn his head aside, loosen his collars and put the bandaged spatula between upper and lower teeth in order not to bite the tongue.

5. Keep the surroundings quiet, reduce stimulation, pay close attention to the change of body temperature, pulse, breath, pupilla, complexion, etc..

Chapter Eight
Arteriosclerotic Cerebral Infarction

This diseas belongs to Zhong Feng (wind stroke) in traditional Chinese medicine.

I. ETIOLOGY AND PATHOGENESIS

Congenital insufficiency or improper care after birth infures the Zang-Fu organs, consumes yin essence, leading to imbalance of yin and yang. Besides, the patient is affected by certain pathogenic factors such as excessive drinking of alcohol, fatigue and excessive emotional change, leading to sudden adverse movement of qi and blood in ascending and descending and obstruction of the channels by phlegm or blood stasis.

II. MAIN POINTS OF DIAGNOSIS

1. The osnet of the disease is abrupt and is usually occurs at night when the patient is taking a rest.

2. Persons over 40 years old have a predilection for the disease.

3. The initial attack is often preceded by some signs such as dizziness, numbness of the limbs, deviation of mouth and stiff tongue, etc..

4. It is often induced by mental depression, overstrain and overstress, ex-

cessive alcohol drinking and voracious eating, etc..

5. The main symptoms are coma and mental confusion, hemiplegia, numbness of the affected side, deviation of mouth and tongue, dysphasia or aphasia.

6. The pulse of the affected side is more wiry and slippery and the tongue coating mostly white and sticky or yellow and dry.

III. DIFFERENTIATION AND
TREATMENT OF COMMON SYNDROMES

1. Sudden Hyperactivity of Liver Yang and Stirring-up of Wind-fire.

Main Symptoms and Signs: hemiplegia, deviation of mouth and tongue, dysphasia or aphasia, numbness of affected side, headache, dizziness, red face and eyes, bitter mouth, dry throat, mental restlessness, irritability, deep yellow urine, dry stool, red or deep red tongue with thin and yellow coating, and wiry and forceful pulse.

Therapeutic Principles: Soothing the liver yang, reducing fire, activating blood circulation and removing obstruction from the channel.

Recipe 1: Ping Gan Xie Huo Tang

Ramulus Uncariae cum Uncis	30 g
Flos Chrysanthemi	10 g
Spica Prunellae	15 g
Cortex Moutan Radicis	15 g
Concha Margaritifera Usta	30 g
Radix Achyranthis Bidentatae	20 g
Radix Paeoniae Rubra	10 g

Decoct the above ingredients in water for oral use.

Recipe 2: Dan Gou Liu Zhi Yin, modified.

Radix Salviae Miltiorrhizae	30-60 g
Ramulus Uncariae cum Uncis (to be decocted later)	15-30 g
Herba Siegesbeckiae	12-24 g
Spica Prunellae	12-24 g

Lumbricus	9 g
Flos Carthami	6 g
Ramulus Mori	15 g
Ramulus Citri Reticulatae	15 g
Ramulus Pini	15 g
Ramulus Persicae	15 g
Ramulus Abies	15 g
Ramulus Bambosae	15 g
Radix Glycyrrhizae	3 g

Decoct the above ingredients in water for oral use.

Modification: In case of preponderance of phlegm, add Fructus Trichosanthis 15 g and Semen Raphani 20 g; in case of coma, Radix Curcumae 9 g and Rhizoma Acori Graminei 9 g; in case of persistent high blood pressure, Ochra Haematitum 30 g and Achyranthis Bidentatae 20 g.

Recipe 3: Li Xiu Lin Shi Fan Wei Jian Zheng Fang

Ochra Haematitum	30 g
Gypsum Firbrosum	30 g
Radix Paeoniae Alba	15 g
Caulis Bambusae in Taeniam	20 g
Exocarpium Citri Grandis	9 g
Rhizoma Acori Graminei	9 g
Poria	30 g
Semen Amomi Cardamomi	3 g
Herba Eupatorii	20 g

Decoct the above ingredients in water for oral use.

Modification: In case of hematemesis and hematochezia, add San Qi Fen (powder of Radix Notoginseng) 3-6 g (to be taken following its infusion), or Yun Nan Bai Yao to be taken following its infusion 0.5 g each time, 4 times daily.

Recipe 4: Ping Gan Huo Xue Tang

Cornu Antelopis	1.5-3 g
Concha Haliotidis	30 g
Ramulus Uncariae cum Uncis	15-30 g
Radix Achyranthis Bidentatae	9-15 g

Rhizoma Ligustici Chuanxiong	9 g
Flos Carthami	9-15 g
Semen Persicae	9 g
Eupolyphaga seu Steleophaga	9 g

Decoct the above ingredients in water for oral use.

Modification: In case of constipation with fullness sensation in the abdomen, add Rhizoma et Rhei 9 g and Fructus Trichosanthis 30 g.

In case of aphasia with thick and sticky tongue coating, add Arisaema cum Bile 9 g and Rhizoma Acori Graminei 9 g.

In case of convulsion, add powder of Scorpio 3-6 g to be taken following its infusion.

In case of mental restlessness, add Calcitum 30 g.

2. Obstruction of the Channels by Wind-phlegm and Blood Stasis.

Main Symptoms and Signs: Hemiplegia, deviation of mouth and tongue, dysphasia or aphasia, numbness of affected side, dizziness and vertigo, dark pale tongue with thin and white or white and sticky coating, and wiry and slippery pulse.

Therapeutic Principles: Dispelling wind, resolving phlegm, activating blood circulation and removing obstruction from the channel.

Recipe 1: Hua Tan Tong Luo Yin

Rhizoma Pinelliae Praeparata	10 g
Rhizoma Atractylodis Macrocephalae	10 g
Rhizoma Gastrodiae	10 g
Arisaema cum Bile	6 g
Radix Salviae Miltiorrhizae	30 g
Rhizoma Cyperi	15 g
Radix et Rhizoma Rhei Praparata	5 g

Decoct the above ingredients in water for oral use.

Recipe 2: Xi Feng Hua Tan Tang, modified.

Poria	12 g
Rhizoma Pinelliae	12 g
Exocarpium Citri Grandis	12 g
Caulis Bambusae in Taeniam	12 g

Rhizoma Acori Graminei	12 g
Rhizoma Arisaema cum Bile Praeparata	12 g
Bombyx Batryticatus	9 g
Ramulus Uncariae cum Uncis	20 g
Scorpio	9 g
Herba Siegesbeckiae	30 g
Semen Persicae	12 g
Flos Carthami	9 g

Decoct the above ingredients in water for oral use.

3. Excess Syndrome of Fu Organ due to Phlegm-heat Complicated with Upward Disturbance of Wind-phlegm.

Main Symptoms and Signs: Hemiplegia, deviation of mouth and tongue, dysphasia or aphasia, numbness of the affected side, abdominal distention, dry stool, constipation, dizziness, vertigo, expectoration with possible profuse sputum, dark red or dark pale tongue with yellow or yellow and sticky coating, and wiry, slippery and full pulse.

Therapeutic Principle: Removing obstruction from the Fu organ and resolving phlegm.

Recipe 1: tong Fu Hua Tan Yin

Radix et Rhizoma Rhei	10 g
Fructus Trichosanthis	30 g
Airsaema cum Bile	6 g
Natrii Sulfas	10 g

Decoct the above ingredients in water for oral use.

Recipe 2: Da huang Gua Lou Tang

Radix et Rhizoma Rhei	6-12 g
Fructus Trichosanthis	15-30 g
Lumbricus	9 g
Eupolyphaga seu Steleophaga	9 g
Semen Sinapis Albaee	9 g

Decoct the above ingredients in water for oral use.

4. Deficiency of Qi with Stasis of Blood

Main Symptoms and Signs: Hemiplegia, deviation of mouth and tongue, dysphasia or aphasia, numbness of the affected region, pallor, shortness of breath, salivation. spontaneous sweating, palpitation, loose stool, distention and swelling of hands and feet, dark pale tongue with thin and white or white and sticky coating, and deep and thready or thready and slow or thready and wiry pulse.

Therapeutic Principle: Tonifying qi and activating blood circulation.

Recipe 1: Yi Qi Huo Xue Tang

Radix Astragali seu Hedysari	30 g
Semen Persicae	10 g
Flos Carthami	10 g
Radix Paeoniae Rubra	20 g
Radix Angelicae Sinensis	10 g
Lumbricus	10 g
Rhizoma Ligustici Chuanxiong	5 g

Decoct the above ingredients in water for oral use.

Recipe 2: bu Yang Huan Wu Tang (Decoction for Invigorating Yang), modified.

Radix Astragali seu hedysari	15-30 g
Rhizoma Ligustici Chuanxiong	6-9 g
Radix Angelicae Sinensis	9-12 g
Radix Paeoniae Rubra	9-12 g
Lumbricus	9-12 g
Semen Persicae	9-12 g
Radix Achyranthis Bidentatae	15 g
Radix Salviae Miltiorrhizae	15-30 g

Decoct the above ingredients in water for oral use.

Recipe 3: Huang Qi Wu Wu Tang (Decoction of Five Drugs Containing Astragali seu Hedysari).

Astragali seu Hedysari	60 g
Radix Paeoniae Alba	15 g
Ramulus Cinnamomi	24 g
Rhizoma Zingiberis Recens	9 g
Fructus Ziziphi Jujubae	5 pieces

Decoct the above ingredients in water for oral use.

Modification: In case of hemiplegia on the left side, add Radix Angelicae Sinensis 30 g; Achyranthis Bidentatae 9 g for paralysis of the lower limbs; Fructus Chaenomelis 15 g for contgracture of the tendons; Os tigris 9 g for weakness of the legs; Radix Aconiti Praeparata 15 g for slow and thready pulse.

5. Stirring-up of Endogenous Wind due to Deficiency of Yin.

Main Symptoms and Signs: Hemiplegia, deviation of mouth and tongue, dsyphasia or aphasia, numbness of the affected side, mental restlessness, insomnia, vertigo, tinnitus, hotness sensation in the palms and soles, deep red or dark red tongue with no or little coating, and thready and wiry or thready, wiry and rapid pulse.

Therapeutic Principles: Nourishing yin and dispelling wind.

Recipe 1: Xi Xian Zhi Yin Tang

Herba Siegesbeckiae Praeparata	50 g
Radix Rehmanniae	15 g
Rhzima Anemarrhenae Praeparata	20 g
Radix Angelica Sinensis	15 g
Fructus Lycii	15 g
Radix Paeoniae Rubra	25 g
Plastrum Testudinis	10 g
Radix Achyranthis Bidentatae	10 g
Flos Chrysanthemi	15 g
Radix Curcumae	15 g
Radix Salviae Miltiorrhizae	15 g
Cortex Phellodendri	5 g

Decoct the above ingredients in water for oral use.

Recipe 3: Yu Yin Xi Feng Tang

Radix Rehmanniae	20 g
Radix Scrophulariae	15 g
Fructus Ligustri Lucidi	15 g
Ramulus Loranthi	30 g
Ramulus Uncariae cum Uncis	30 g
Radix Paeoniae Alba	20 g

Radix Salviae Miltiorrhizae	15 g

Decoct the above ingredients in water for oral use.

6. Block of the Mind by Phlegm-Heat

Main Symptoms and Signs: Abrupt onset of coma or mental confusion with snoring, rattle in the throat, hemiplegia, contracture of limbs, neck rigidity, fever, restlessness, convulsion of the limbs, deep red tongue with brownish yellow, dry and sticky coating, and wiry, slippery and rapid pulse.

Therapeutic Principles: Clearing away heat, resolving phlegm and opening the mind.

Recipe: Ling Jiao Gou Teng Tang (Decoction of Cornu Saigae Tataricae and Uncariae cum Uncis), modified.

Cornu Antelopis	4.5 g
Concha Haliotidis	30 g
Os Draconis	30 g
Concha Ostreae	30 g
Radix Paeoniae Alba	30 g
Ramulus Uncariae cum Uncis	15 g
Radix Achyranthis Bidentatae	15 g
Radix Rehmanniae	30 g
Spica Prunellae	15 g
Cortex Moutan Radicis	9 g

Decoct the above ingredients in water for oral use.

7. Mist of the Mind due to Phlegm-Damp

Main Symptoms and Signs: The patient has constitutional deficiency of yang with accumulation of phlegm-damp in the interior. During the attack, there are coma, hemiplegia, cold and flaccid limbs, pallor, dark lips, profuse phlegm, dark pale tongue with white and sticky tongue coating, and deep and slippery or deep and slow pulse.

Therapeutic Principle: Dispelling wind, resolving phlegm and opening the mind.

1) Recipe

Rhizoma Arisaematis Praeparata	12 g
Rhizoma Pinelliae Praeparata	12 g

Fructus Citri Aurantii Immaturus	9 g
Pericarpium Citri Reticulatae	9 g
Rhizoma Acori Graminei	6 g
Poria	9 g
Rhizoma Zingiberis	6 g
Radix Ginseng	3 g
Radix Glycyrrhizae	3 g
Succus Bambusae	30 g

Decoct the above ingredients in water twice to obtain 300 ml of decoction to be taken together with one pill of Su He Xiang Wan through oral or nasal feeding. One or two doses daily.

2) In severe case or no good therapeutic effect is obtained, take Calculus Macacae 0.3 g together with the above decoction.

8. Exhaustion of Primordial Qi and Scatter of Mind

Main Symptoms and Signs: Sudden coma or mental confusion, flaccidity of limbs with hands relaxed, cold limbs, profuse sweating, and clammy body in severe case, incontinenceof bowel movement and micturition, flaccid tongue which is dark purple with white and sticky coating, and deep and slow or deep and fading pulse.

Therapeutic Principles: Tonify Primordial qi, restoring yang and saving the patient from collapse.

Recipe: Shen Fu Tang (Decoction of Ginseng and Aconiti)

Radix Ginseng	30 g
Radix Aconiti Praeparata	9 g

Decoct the above ingredients in water twice to obtain 200 ml of decoction to be taken through frequent oral or nasal feeding.

Chapter Nine
Hypertensive Cerebral Hemorrhage

According to its clinical manifestations, hypertensive cerebral hemorrhage corresponds to apoplexy in which the Zang organs are attacked.

I. ETIOLOGY AND PATHOGENESIS

Fundamentally, the patient has imbalance of Yin and Yang in which Yin is insufficient in the lower and Yang hyperactive in the upper due to congenital deficiency or improper care after birth. Besides, the patient is affected by invasion of exogenous pathogenic factors, excessive emotional changes, improper work and rest or irregular food-intake which lead to adverse movement of qi and blood in ascending and descending, and extravasation of blood, giving rise to sudden attack of apoplexy.

II. MAIN POINTS OF DIAGNOSIS

1. This disease usually abruptly occurs during emotional excitement or physical exertion with sudden coma and fall.

2. It happens more often in cases over 40 years old.

3. Most of the patients have the history of headache, vertigo or hypertension which gets worse before the stroke with such signs as temperal aphasia, numbness of the limbs, and blurred vision. the attack is often induced by invasion of exogenous pathogenous factors, excitement, voracious eating and alcohol drinking, and fatigue.

4. The main clinical manifestations are sudden fall and unconsciousness, hemiplegia, deviation of mouth and tongue, dsyphasia or even aphasia.

5. Cerebrospinal fluid presents a bloody color and the hemorrhagic focus can be found during a CT scan.

III. DIFFERENTIATION AND
TREATMENT OF COMMON SYNDROMES

1. Attack of the Brain by Wind-Fire

Main Symptoms and Signs: The patient often has headache, dizziness and vertigo with excessive emotional change, voracious alcohol drinking or over strain and stress. The pathological condition may suddenly change, giving rise to such manifestations as trance, semiconsciousness, hemiplegia, rigidity or contracture of the limbs, dry stool or constipation, deep red tongue with yellow sticky and dry coating, and wiry, slippery, full and rapid pulse.

Therapeutic Principle: Dispelling wind, reducing fire, resolving phlegm and opening the mind.

1) An Gong Niu Huang Wan (Bolus of Calculus Bovis for Resurrection) to be dissolved in water for oral application or nasal feeding, one pill every 6 hours during the first 3 days, and one pill every 12 hours during the next 4 days.

2) An Gong Niu Huang San (Powder of Calculus Bovis for Resurrection) to be taken following its infusion or by nasal feeding 1.6 g each time, once or twice daily.

3) Add 40-60 ml of Qing Kai Ling to 250 ml of 5% glucose solution for intravenous drip, once a day.

4) Experienced recipe:

Scorpio	3 g
Concretio Silicea Bambusae	5 g
Cornu Antelopis	3 g
Margarita	0.5 g

Grind the above ingredients into fine powder which is divided into 3-4 portions. To be taken following its infusion or by nasal feeding separately. One dose daily.

5) Experienced recipe:

Cornu Antelopis	4.5 g
Concha Haliotidis	30 g
Plastrum Testudinis	30 g
Os Draconis	30 g
Radix Praeoniae Alba	30 g
Ramulus Uncariae cum Uncis	15 g
Radix Achyranthis Bidentatae	15 g
Radix Rehmanniae 7 30 g	
Cortex Moutan Radicis	9 g
Spica Prunellae	15 g

Decoct the above ingredients in water twice to obtain 300 ml of decoction. To be taken separately in the morning, at noon and in the evening orally or by nasal feeding.

6) Take Bai Yao orally or by nasal feeding 0.5 g each time, once every 4 hours during the first 3-4 days, once every 6 hours during the 5th-10th days, and 3 times a day during the 11th-14th days.

2. Mist of the Mind by Phlegm-Damp

Main Symptoms and Signs: The patient has constitutional insufficiency of Yang with accumulation of phlegm-damp in the interior. After the attack of the disease, there may be coma, hemiplegia, flaccidity of the limbs, or even cold limbs, pale complexion, dark lips, preponderance of phlegm, dark pale tongue with white and sticky coating, and deep and slippery or deep and slow pulse.

Therapeutic Principle: Resolving phlegm and opening the mind.

Recipe: Di Tan Tang, modified.

Rhizoma Arisaematis Praeparata	12 g
Rhizoma Pinelliae Praeparata	12 g
Fructus Citri Aurantii Immaturus	9 g
Pericarpium Citri Reticulatae	9 g
Rhizoma Acori Graminei	6 g
Poria	9 g

Rhizoma Zingiberis	3 slices
Radix Ginseng	3 g
Radix Glycyrrhizae	30 g

Decoct the above ingredients in water twice to obtain 250 ml of decoction. To be taken for 3 times through oral or nasal feeding, one to two doses a day.

Modification: In case of critical condition or if no good therapeutic result is obtained, Su He Xiang Wan (one pill each time) or Hou Zao San (3 g each time) could be taken together with the above decoction once or twice daily.

3. Block of the Mind by Phlegm-Heat

Main Symptoms and Signs: Abrupt onset with coma or mental confusion, snoring, rattle in the throat, ehmiplegia, rigity and contracture of the limbs, stiffness of the neck, fever, restlessness, or even cold extremities, frequent convulsion, occasional hematemesis, deep red tongue with brownish yellow, dry and sticky coating, and wiry, slippery and rapid coating.

Therapeutic Principle: Clearing away heat, resolving phlegm, dispelling wind and opening the mind.

Recipe: Chang Pu Yu Jin Tang (Decoction of Acori Graminei and Curcumae), modified.

Rhizoma Acori Graminei	12 g
Radix Curcumae	12 g
Fructus Gardeniae	9 g
Succus Bambosae	30 ml
cortex Moutan Radicis	12 g
Folium Bambosae	3 g
Fructus Firsythiae	9 g
Arisaema cum Bile	6 g
Concretio Silicea Bambusae	6 g
Cornu Antelopis	1.5 g

Decoct the above ingredients in water twice to obtain 200 ml of decoction to be taken through oral or nasal feeding for several times, one dose a day.

Modification: In case of severe coma, add Zhi Bao Dan or An Gong Niu Huang Wan, one pill each time and once or twice a day, or grind Scorpio 3 g, Concretio Silicea bambosae 5 g, Powder of Cornu Antelopis 3 g and Margarita 0.

5 g together into fine powder. To be taken through oral or nasal feeding for 3-4 times, once every 6-8 hours.

4. Exhaustion of Primordial Qi and Scatter of the Mind

Main Symptoms and Signs: Sudden coma, mental confusion, flaccidity of the limbs, cold limbs with sweating, and in severe case, clammy body, incontenence of bowel movement and micturition, flaccid tongue which is dark purple with white and sticky coating, and deep and slow or deep and weak pulse.

Therapeutic Principles: Tonifying qi, restoring yang, strengthening the anti-pathogenic qi and saving the patient from collapse.

Recipe: Shen Fu Tang (Decoction of Ginseng and Aconiti), modified.

Radix Ginseng	15 g
Radix Aconiti Praeparata	15 g
Radix Ophiopogonis	30 g

Decoct the above ingredients in water twice to obtain 150- 200 ml of decoction. To be taken through oral or nasal feeding for 3 to 4 times.

Modification: In case of persistent hiccup, add Haematitum 30 g and Rhizoma et Radix Rhei 6 g; in case of persistent profuse sweating, Os Draconis 20 g, Concha Ostreae 20 g, Fructus Corni 12 g and Fructus Schisandrae 6 g. Decoct the above ingredients in water and take the decoction through nasal feeding for 3-4 times; in case of hematemesis, Bai Yao 0.5-1 g (to be taken following its infusion); in case of convulsion, grind Scorpio 3 g and powder of Cornu Antelopis 1.5 g into fine powder to be taken twice following its infusion.

Chapter Ten
Migraine

Migraine corresponds to Nao Feng (headache caused by pathogenic wind), Shou Feng (headache caused by pathogenic wind) and Tou Feng Tou Tong (headache caused by attack of the head by pathogenic wind) in traditional Chinese medicine.

I. ETIOLOGY AND PATHOGENESIS

Congenital deficiency or lack of proper care after birth leads to injuries of Zang-fu orans and imbalance of yin and yang, which are complicated with invasion of exogenous pathogenic factors or excessive emotional changes or fatigue, resulting in reversed flow of qi and blood and malnutrition of the brain, giving rise to abrupt attack of headache with intermittent pain.

II. MAIN POINTS OF DIAGNOSIS

1. This disease is usually related to inheritance, and may occur repeatedly with the first attack at childhood.

2. It is often induced by seasonal pathogenic factors, overfatigue, tension, excitement, poor sleep or menstrual period.

3. The patient may have such symptoms and signs before attacks as lethargy, spiritlessness or hyperhedoma, blurred vision, photophobia, and possiblly blind spot, hemianopsia, distention and pain of the eyeballs, or abnormal sensation of the limbs, or kinetic disturbance, etc..

4. There are repeated attacks of intolerable burning throbbing or boring pain on the forehead, temple and occiput unilaterally in most cases and bilaterally in

few cases. The pain usually lasts for few minutes or even 1-2 days. Sometimes it attacks several times a day. It may reattack in few months or few years.

5. It is often accompanied by nausea, vomiting, abdominal distention, diarrhea, polyhidrosis, lacrimation, pallor, bluish purple skin and edema, etc..

III. DIFFERENTIATION AND
TREATMENT OF COMMON SYNDROMES

1. Obstruction of the Collaterals by Stagnation of Wind and Phlegm and Blood Stasis.

Main Symptoms and Signs: Intermittent headache which is aggravated by wind and cold, no thirst, thin and white tongue coating, and superficial, wiry and tense pulse.

Therapeutic Principle: Dispelling wind, resolving phlegm, activating blood circulation and arresting pain.

Recipe 1: San Pian Tang, modified.

Rhizoma Ligustici Chuanxiong	30 g
Radix Angelicae Dahuricae	15 g
Radix Paeoniae Alba	15 g
Semen Sinapis Alba	9 g
Rhizoma Cyperi	6 g
Radix bupleuri	3 g
Semen Pruni	3 g
Radix Glycyrrhizae	3 g

Decoct the above ingredients in water twice to obtain 300 ml of decoction. To be taken half in the morning and half in the evening while it is warm, one dose daily.

Recipe 2: Chuanxiong Ding Tong Tang (Decoction of Ligustici Chuanxiong for Relieving Pain), modified.

Rhizoma Ligustici Chuanxiong	30 g
Radix Paeoniae Rubra	15 g

Radix Salviae Miltiorrhizae	30 g
Radix Ledebouriellae	12 g
Herba Asari	6 g
Radix Aconiti	6 g
Semen Sinapis Albae	15 g
Semen Coicis	30 g
Fructus Amomi	9 g

Decoct the above ingredients in water for oral dose.

The following prescription be used to prevent reattacks.

Rhizoma Ligustici Chuanxiong	15 g
Radix Angelicae Sinensis	9 g
Flos Carthami	9 g
Radix Angelicae Dahuricae	9 g
Fructus Tribuli	9 g
Flos Chrysanthemi	9 g
Ramulus Uncariae cum Uncis	6 g
Concha Margaritifera Usta	30 g

Decoct the above ingredients in water for oral use.

2. Flaring-up of Wind-Fire

Main Symptoms and Signs: Sudden attack of bursting or stabbing headache, red face with sweating, thirst, mental restlessness, red tongue with thin and yellow coating, and wiry and rapid pulse.

Therapeutic Principles: Dispelling wind-heat, removing obstruction from the channel and arresting pain.

Recipe: Qing Shang Juan Tong Tang

Radix Ophiopogonis	15 g
Radix Scutellariae	12 g
Fructus Viticis	12 g
Flos Chrysanthemi	12 g
Rhizoma seu Radix Notopterygii	9 g
Radix Ledebouriellae	9 g
Rhizoma Atractylodis	9 g
Radix Angelicae Sinensis	9 g

Radix Angelicae Dahuricae	9 g
Rhizoma Ligustici Chuanxiong	15 g
Herba Asari	6 g
Radix Glycyrrhizae	3 g

Decoct the above ingredients in water for oral use.

Modification: In case of left migraine, add Flos Carthami 9 g, Radix Bupleuri 9 g, Radix Gentianae 12 g and Radix Rehmanniae 9 g; in case of right migraine, Rhizoma Gastrodiae 12 g, Rhizoma Pinelliae 12 g, Fructus Crataegi 12 g and Fructus Citri Aurantii Immaturus 12 g; in case of vertex headache, Rhizoma Ligustici 9 g, Rhizoma et Radix Rhei 6 g and Herba Schizonepetae 9 g; in case of headache caused by invasion of the brain by pathogenic wind complicated with nasal obstruction or turbid nasal discharge, Fructus Xanthii 12 g, Fructus Chaenomelis 9 g and Herba Schizonepetae 9 g; in case of headache caused by deficiency of qi and blood, Radix Astragali seu Hedysari 15 g, Radix Ginseng 9 g or Radix Pseudostellariae 30 g, Radix Paeoniae Rubra 12 g, Radix Paeoniae 12 g, Radix Rehmanniae 12 g and Radix Rehmanniae Praeparata 12 g, or use Quanxie Gouteng San (Powder of Scorpio and Uncaria cum Uncis), modified.

Scorpio	6 pieces
Ramulus Uncariae cum Uncis	9 g
Radix Ginseng Rubra	6 g
Radix Angelicae Dahuricae	9 g
Radix Aconiti Praeparata	6 g

Administration: Bake the above ingredients together, grind them into fine powder which is divided into 9 equal portions. Put one portion of the powder into 250 ml of boiling water and cover it tightly for 20 minutes. Then, remove the residue and drink the juice. Take the above medicinal juice 3 times a day.

In case of attack during menstrual period, Yang Jiao Chong Ji may be used.

Cornu Antelopis	3 g
Rhizoma Ligustici Chuanxiong	6 g
Radix Angelicae Dahuricae	9 g
Radix Aconiti Praeparata	6 g

Administration: Grind the above ingredients together into fine powder which is divided into 2 equal portions. Put one portion in a cup with 250 ml of boiling water, cover it tightly for 30 minutes, and then take away the residue and drink the juice while it is warm. Such administration is taken once in the morning and once in the evening and 10 days are considered as one course.

Zhi Tong San (Powder for Relieving Pain) can also be be used:

Borneolum Syntheticum	3 g
Natrii Sulfas	6 g
Moschus	0.5 g
Menthol	2 g

Administration: Grind the above ingredients together into fine powder which is put in a bottle tightly closed during an attack of migraine, wrap 0.3 g of the powder in a small piece of gauze and then put it in the nostril of opposite side, that is, left nostril for right migraine and right nostril for left. This method is indicated in various kinds of headache and can obtain immediate effect.

Chapter Eleven
Sudden Deafness

Sudden deafness, a sensorineural hearing loss, occurs abruptly for reasons unkown. Its main clinical feature is a sudden profound sensorineural deafness, accompanied by tinnitus and dizziness and a tendency to get cured spontaneously. The disorder is usually unilateral and occurs more often in females and mostly in the middle-aged. In TCM, it belongs to the category of "Bao Long" or "Cu Long", both meaning sudden deafness.

I. MAIN POINTS OF DIAGNOSIS

1. In some cases there exist mental factors or a history of virus infection prior to the attack of the disease.

2. It occurs abruptly. The patient often has severe deafness or even loses hearing entirely within an hour or one day.

3. There is often an accompanying tinnitus or vertigo.

4. Optic endoscopy examination indicates normal.

5. Audiometric curve shows that the deafness is a sensorineural hearing loss. Low-frequency deafness and even deafness are seen more often and recruitment may be present.

II. DIFFERENTIATION AND TREATMENT
OF COMMON SYNDROMES

Main Symptoms and Signs: Deafness and tinnitus suddenly occur, in most cases resulting from tense mood or overwork, and are accompanied with restlessness, irritability, dizziness, and insomnia. The tongue is light red with little fur. The puls eis taut.

Therapeutic Principles: Promoting the flow of qi and blood circulation, relaxing muscles and tendons and removing obstruction from the channels.

Recipe: Decoction for Activating Blood Circulation with additional drugs

Semen Persicae	9 g
Flos Carthami	9 g
Rhizoma Ligustici Chuanxiong	9 g
Rhizoma Acori Graminei	9 g
Radix Bupleuri	9 g
Radix Paeoniae Rubra	15 g
Radix Puerariae	30 g
Rhizoma Zingiberis Recens	6 g
Fructus Ziziphi Jujubae	7 pcs
Moschus	20 mg

For those who have a feeling of fullness and discomfort in the chest and hypochondrium as well as restlessness and irritability, add 9 grams of gentian root , 9 grams of scutellaria root and 15 grams of capejasmine fruit. For those with severe tinnitus, add 30 grams of magnetite which is to be decocted first and 9 grams of chastetree fruit. For those with dizziness, add 30 grams of fleece-flower stem, 9 grams of gastrodia tuber and 30 grams of abalone shell.

Chapter Twelve
Infectious Polyradiculitis

Infectius polyradiculitis, also called Guillain-Barre syndrome, is an inflammatory disease of nerve roots characterized by symmetric flaccid paralysis of limbs. It is often caused by general viral and bacterial infections or intoxication. This disease belongs to the category of "Wei Zheng" (flaccidity syndrome) in traditional Chinese medicine.

I. MAIN POINTS OF DIAGNOSIS

1. Ther may be histories of prodromal infection about 2 weeks before the appearance of nervous symptoms, such as upper respiratory tract infection, rubella, mumps, diarrhea, etc. .

2. The early symptoms include irritating pain and paresthesia of the nerve root. This gradually results in general sensational damage, including loss of the senses of pain, touch, temperature, locality and vibration. When the involvement of distal limbs-hands and feet occurs, it is often manifested as a "glove and stocking anesthesia". Paralysis of cranial nerve and paralysis of respiratory muscles may be present, the latter can produce dyspnea or respiratory failure in severe cases. These often appear with symptoms of vergetative nerve functional disturbance, such as hyperhidrosis or hypohidrosis, cold extremities, flush, transient retention or incontinence of urine, constipation or diarrhea. Loss or diminution of tendon reflexes, weakness and muscular atrophy are usually present during the course of the disease.

3. Laboratory examinations reveal elevated leukocyte and erythrocyte sedimentation rate. Cerebrospinal fluid (CSF) changes are of value in making diagnosis. The protein in CSF becomes elevated but white cell count in CSF is normal

one to two weeks after the onset of clinical manifestation. This feature is called "isolation phenomenon of cell-protein" and can persist for several months till convalescence.

II. DIFFERENTIATION AND TREATMENT OF COMMON SYNDROMES

1. Obstruction of the Channels and Collaterals by Damp-heat

Main Symptoms and Signs: Flaccid paralysis of extremities, especially symmetrical paralysis of lower limbs, accompanied with heavy sensation of the body, oppressed feeling in the chest, dysphoria with smothery sensation, difficult diarrhea, scanty yellow urine, red tip and margin of the tongue with yellow and greasy fur, soft or soft and rapid pulse.

Therapeutic Principle: Removing pathogenic heat and dampness.

Recipe: Three Wonderful Drugs Powder with additional herbs.

Rhizoma Atractylodis	9 g
Cortex Phellodendri	9 g
Radix Achyranthis Bidentatae	9 g
Semen Coicis	15 g
Rhizoma Dioscoreae Septemlobae	9 g
Radix Gentianae Macrophyllae	9 g

All the above drugs are to be decocted in water for oral administration. In the presence of impairment of yin by damp- heat, manifested as feverish sensation in the feet, and dry tongue, the following drugs should be added: rehmannia root 9 g, scrophularia root 9 g, and dendrobium 9 g.

2. Deficiency of the Liver-yin and Kidney-yin

Main Symptoms and Signs: Long-standing malady with muscular strophy, deformity of the limbs, aching and weakness of the back and loin, red tongue without fur, and thready and rapid pulse.

Therapeutic Principles: Nourishing and invigorating the liver-yin and kidney-yin.

Recipe: Modified Huqian Bolus

Cortex Phellodendri	9 g
Palstrum Testudinis	9 g
Rhizoma Anemarrhenae	6 g
Radix Rehmanniae Praeparata	9 g
Pericarpium Citri Reticulatae	6 g
Radix Paeoniae Alba	9 g
Herba Cynomorii	9 g
Rhizoma Zingiberis	3 g
Colla Cornu Cervi	3 g
Semen Cuscutae	12 g
Fructus Mori	9 g

All the above drugs are to be decocted in water for oral administration.

3. Deficiency of both Qi and Blood

Main Symptoms and Signs: Pale complexion, lassitude, disinclination to talk due to deficiency of qi, abnormal stool, flaccidity of the limbs, no warm feeling of the face, pale tongue with thin and white fur, and slow and weak pulse.

Therapeutic Principles: Invigorating qi and nourishing blood.

Recipe: Modified Decoction of Eight Precious Ingredients

Radix Codonopsis Pilosulae	9 g
Radix Astragali seu Pilosulae	12 g
Rhizoma Atractylodis Macrocephalae	9 g
Poria	12 g
Radix Angelicae Sinensis	9 g
Radix Paeoniae Rubra	9 g
Radix Paeoniae Alba	9 g
Rhizoma Ligustici Chuanxiong	6 g
Radix Rehmanniae Praeparata	9 g
Ramulus Cinnamomi	6 g
Radix Achyranthis Bidentatae	9 g
Radix Glycyrrhizae	3 g
Fructus Chaenomelis	9 g

All the above drugs are to be decocted in water for oral administration.

In case of deficiency of the spleen-yang, marked by cold limbs and aversion to cold, the following drugs should be added: prepared aconite root 9 g, dodder seed 9 g, desertliving cistanche 9 g and epimedieum 9 g.

Chapter Thirteen
Trigeminal Neuralgia

This disease is more or less included in Tou Feng Tou Tong (headche caused by attack of the head by pathogenic wind) and Pian Tou Tong (migraine) in traditional Chinese medicine.

I. ETIOLOGY AND PATHOGENESIS

Attack of the head by pathogenic wind leads to stagnation of the blood and obstruction of the channel, giving rise to pain. Since pathogenic wind is characterized by constant movement and rapid change, the occurrence of this disease is abrupt with intermittent pain.

II. MAIN POINTS OF DIAGNOSIS

1. It is characterized by paroxysmal burning sensation on the face with severe flash pain accompanied with facial spasm and lacrimation which usually last for few seconds and then relieves spontaneously. The patient feels nothing abnormal during interval of attacks.

2. the pain is usually induced by muscular movement of the face and referred to the lips, ala nasi and jaw.

3. Generally, there is no positive symptoms of nerve system.

4. Clinically, it should be differentiated from toothache, sinusitis and glossopharyngeal neuralgia.

III. DIFFERENTIATION AND
TREATMENT OF COMMON SYNDROMES

1. Invasion of Exogenous Pathogenic Wind-Heat

Main Symptoms and Signs: Paroxysmal burning stabbing pain on one side of the face which is accompanied usually by fever, thirst, sore throat, thin and yellow tongue coating, and wiry and rapid pulse.

Therapeutic Principles: Dispelling pathogenic wind and heat, removing obstruction from the channel and arresting pain.

Recipe: Xiong Zhi Shigao Tang (Decoction of Ligustici Chuanxiong, Angelica Dahuricae and Gypsum Fibrosum), modified.

Rhizoma Ligustici Chuanxiong	20 g
Gypsum Fibrosum	30 g
Flos Chrysanthemi	9 g
Herba Menthae	9 g
Lumbricus	9 g
Fructus Arctii	12 g
Radix Angelica Dahuricae	12 g
Rhizoma Phragmitis	30 g

Decoct the above ingredients in water for oral use.

Application of acupuncture in combination with needling the subsequent points:

Tinggong(SI19), Xiaguan(ST7), Hegu(LI4), Sibai(ST2), Yuyao(EX-HN4).

2. Invasion of Exogenous Pathogenic Wind-Cold

Main Symptoms and Signs: Severe pain, aversion to cold, fever, thin and white tongue-coating, and wiry and tense pulse.

Therapeutic Principles: Dispelling cold and arresting pain.

Recipe: Chuan Xiong Cha Tiao San (Powder of Ligustici Chuanxiong mixed with Camelliae Sinensis), modified.

Rhizoma Ligustici Chuanxiong	30 g
Radix Angelica Dahuricae	12 g

Rhizoma seu Radix Notopterygii	12 g
Radix Ledebouriellae	12 g
Herba Asari	6 g
Herba Schizonepetae	6 g
Herba Menthae	6 g
Radix Aconiti Kusnezoffii Praeparata	9 g
Radix glycyrrhizae	6 g

Decoct the above ingredients in water for oral dose.

Modification: In case of severe pain or no significant therapeutic effect after taking the above decoction, add Scolopendra 6 pieces and Scorpio 6 g which are charred by baking and then ground into fine powder to be taken with warm boiled water.

Application of acupuncture in combination with needling Pt. Touwei(ST8), Lieque(LU7), Jiache(ST6), Xiaguan(ST7), Hegu(LI4), etc. may obtain even better result.

3. Obstruction of the Channels by Stasis of Blood.

Main Symptoms and Signs: Repeated attack of fixed stabbing pain, tinnitus, deafness, dark red tongue with possible stagnant spots, and thready and hesitant pulse.

Therapeutic Principles: Activating blood circulation, dispersing blood stasis and arresting pain.

Recipe: tong Qiao Zhi Tong Tang (Decoction for Relieving Pain), modified.

Rhizoma Ligustici Chuanxiong	30 g
Radix Paeoniae Rubra	15 g
Semen Persicae	15 g
Flos Carthami	9 g
Rhizoma Zingiberis	3 slices
Bulbus Allii Fistulosi	1 decimetre
Mochus	0.2 g

Decoct the above ingredients in water for oral use.

Chapter Fourteen
Intercostal Neuralgia

The disease is characterized by prickling or lancinating pain from the distribution region of the intercostal nerve, pertaining to the category of "hypochondriac pain" in traditional Chinese medicine.

I. DIFFERENTIATION

1. Liver-qi depression: Distending pain in the chest and hypochondrium with unfixed localization, slightly alleviated by belching and aggravated by sadness, thin and white tongue coating, taut pulse.

2. Blood stagnation: Fixed stabbing pain in the hypochondriac region, intensified by pressure and at night, alleviated in daytime, dark purplish tongue, sometimes with petechiae or ecchymoses, deep and uneven pulse.

II. TREATMENT

1. Body acupuncture

Prescription: Zhigou(SJ6), Yanglingquan(GB34) and Huatuojiaji points of the corresponding segments.

Supplementary points: For liver-qi depression, Xingjian (LR2) and Taichong(LR3) are added; for blood stagnation, Geshu(BL17), Ganshu(BL18) and Qimen(LR14).

Method: Use filiform needles to puncture the points with reducing method.

2. Auricular acupuncture

Prescription: Xiong (AH10) chest, Shenmen (TF4) shenmen, Jiaogan (AH6a) sympathetic nerve, Zhen(AT3) occiput and Fei(CO14) lung.

Method: Use twirling and rotating method. Give a strong stimulation to the points, and retain the needles for 15 to 30 minutes or so.

Chapter Fifteen
Sciatica

Sciatica refers to the pain in the passage ways of the sciatic nerve and its distribution region, radiating from the buttock along the posterior part of the thigh and the posterolateral portion of the shank to the distal portion. It is mainly caused by sciatic neuritis and the changes of the adjacent structures, belonging to the categories of "Bi Zheng" (arthralgia-syndrome) and "Yao Tui Tong" (pain in the waist and lower extemities) in traditional Chinese medicine.

I. MAIN SYMPTOMS AND SIGNS

At the beginning of the disease, there is usually a lateral pain in the waist and with the development of the disease the pain radiates suddenly or gradually along the buttock of the affected side, the posterior aspect of the thigh and the posterolateral side of the leg and the dorsum of the foot or the lateral margin of foot. And a burning, lancinating or electric- shock like pain may appear along the spreading area of the sciatic nerve. At the beginning, the pain is mostly paroxysmal, increases after tiredness, disappears after rest, and becomes severe and continuous gradually afterwards. Usually there is septal repeated attack which may last several weeks, several months or even several years. On examination, the physiological curvature of the lumbar vertebrae can be seen as flat and straight, or the lateral curvature and the lumbar muscle may look tense. And near the spinous process of the affected side of the lumbar vertebrae there is a distinct tenderness point which radiates towards the lower limbs of the affected side. The test of straight leg-raising is positive. Neck flexion and neck pressure test are also positive. In a long-standing case, there may be hypoesthesia or anesthesia or muscular atrophy of the affected limb.

II. TYPES OF SYNDROMES

1. Arthralgia-Syndrome due to Wind-Cold-Dampness

Pain in the waist and lower extremities, inability to bend, stretch, toss or turn which is aggravated in overcast and rainy weather, heaviness, numbness and cold sensation of the affected region, whitish greasy coating of the tongue, taut pulse.

2. Deficiency of the Liver and Kidney

Pain in the waist and lower extremities, soreness and weakness of the waist and knees, pain and numbness of the affected region, listlessness, thin whitish coating of the tongue, deep thready and feeble pulse.

3. Obstruction of the Channels and Collaterals by Trauma

Obvious traumatic history, drastic pain in the waist and lower extremities with activity disturbance, obvious local tenderness, ecchymoses on the tongue with thin whitish coating, taut and uneven pulse.

III TREATMENT BY ACUPUNCTURE

1. Body Acupuncture

Prescription: Dachangshu(BL25), Shenshu(BL23), Huatuojiaji point on the lumbar region, Ciliao(BL32), Weizhong(BL40), Yanglingquan(GB34) and Juegu(GB39).

Supplementary points: For wind-cold-damp arthralgia, Dazhui(DU14) and Yinlingquan(SP9) are added; for deficiency of the kidney-essence, Pangguangshu(BL28) and Taixi(KI3); for blood stasis obstructing collaterals, Shuigou (DU26) and points which reveal tenderness on palpation.

Method: Use filiform needles to puncture the points with reinforcing or even movement method.

2. Auricular Acupuncture

Prescription: Zuogushenjing (AH6) sciatic nerve, Tun (AH7) gluteus, Yaodizhui(AH9) lumbosacral vertebrae, Shenmen(TF4) shenmen and Pizhixia (AT4) subcortex.

Method: Select 2-3 points for each treatment. Give a moderate and strong stimulation to the points. Retain the needles for 30 minutes. Give the treatment once a day. The seed-embedding therapy is also applicable.

3. Eletrotherapy

Prescription: Jiaji(EX-B2) on the lumbar region, Yanglingquan(GB34) and Weizhong(BL40).

Method: Insert the needles into the points. After arrival of qi, electrify them for 20 minutes with a dense wave or a sparse-dense wave. Give the treatment once daily.

IV. THERAPEUTIC METHODS BY PRACTISING QIGONG

1. Self-Treatment by Practising Qigong

1) Basic Maneuvers

It is advisable to practise Waist Qigong and Lower Limbs Qigong.

2) Auxiliary Maneuvers

(1) Arthralgia due to wind-cold-dampness: It is advisable to practise Eight-Section Brocade and Six-Section Brocade.

(2) Deficiency of the liver and kidney: It is advisable to practise the method of strengthening the kidney and conducting qi in Regulating-Kidney Qigong as well as the method of soothing the liver and conducting qi in Regulating-Liver Qigong.

(3) Obstruction of the channels and collaterals by traumata: It is advisable

to practise Conducting Qigong to raise and lower yin and yang

2. External Qi Therapy

(1) Press and knead Shenshu(BL23), Mingmen(DU4), Yaoyangguan (DU3), Huantiao(GB30), Yanglingquan(GB34), Weizhong(BL40), Chengshan(BL57), Kunlun(BL60) and Taixi(KI3).

(2) Deficiency of the Liver and Kidney: Apply the flat-palm form, use the pulling and rotating manipulations to emit qi onto Shenshu(BL23), Mingmen (DU4), and conduct the channel qi along the Urinary Bladder Meridian to the lower limbs.

(3) Apply flat-palm form, use the pushing, pulling, and leading manipulations to emit qi onto Huantiao(GB30) and conduct qi to the lower limbs so as to make qi balanced.

2) Auxiliary Maneuvers

(1) Arthralgia-syndrome due to wind-cold-dampness: Add the heatstyle conducting-qi method, apply the flat-palm form, use the pulling and leading manipulations to pull the pathogenic qi along the channel out of the body.

(2) Deficiency of the liver and kidney: Apply the flat-palm form, use pulling and rotating manipulations to emit qi onto Shenshu(BL23), Mingmen (DU4) and Guanyuan(RN4).

(3) Obstruction of the channels and collaterals by trauma: Apply flat-palm form, use rotating and leading manipulations to conduct the channel qi along the channels and make use of the wrenching and rocking manipulations.

V. THERAPEUTIC METHODS BY CHINESE MASSAGE

Massage therapy of this disease may produce obvious curative effect in most cases. A secondary case should be treated comprehensively by integrating with the manipulation of massage for the primary case. In addition, a careful differential diagnosis is needed and the massage therapy is forbidden in sciatica caused by tumor, metastatic carcinoma, tuberculosis, etc..

1. Manipulation: Digital-pressing, pressing, kneading, rolling and traction.

2. Points Selection: Dachangshu (BL25), Zhibian (BL54), Huantiao (GB30), Chengfu(BL36), Yinmen(BL37), Liangqiu(ST34), Yanglingquan (GB34), Chengshan(BL57), Jiexi(ST41), Kunlun(BL60).

3. Operation

1) The doctor stands at the affected side of the patient who is in prone position and then applies rolling manipulation for 3 to 5 times to the lumbar muscle of the affected side of the lower lumbar vertebrae and along the posterior aspect of the affected thigh and the posterolateral part of the leg softly at first and then hard and deeply.

2) Then the doctor, with the thumbs overlapped press-kneads the points revealed pain on the waist and the buttock for one to two minutes repeatedly with a bit more strength.

3) Using his elbow, the doctor presses the points of Dachangshu(BL25) and Huantiao(GB30) and the points revealed pain on the waist and the buttock.

4) The doctor digit-presses the points of Chengfu(BL36), Yinmen(BL37), Weizhong(BL40), Chengshan(BL57), Kunlun(BL60), etc..

5) The doctor holds the lumbus and pulls it backwards, once for the right and once for the left.

6) Repeat Operation 1) twice to 3 times.

7) The patient is in prone position, while the doctor, digit-presses to stimulate the points of Futu(ST32), Liangqiu(ST34), Zusanli(ST36), Yanglingquan (GB34), Xuanzhong(GB39) and Jiexi(ST41). Then the doctor rolls from the upper part to the lower part and repeats the operation twice to 3 times.

8) Ask the patient to flex his knee and hip bone. Then the doctor, with one hand grasping the foot sole, the other supporting the affected knee, makes the patient do compulsory flexion of the hip bone, stretch the knee and extend the ankle, twice to 3 times. Be sure that the stretching angle of the lower limb should be within the limits of the patient's movement.

9) Let the patient's lower limb stretch straight and accomplish the operation with the manipulation of foulaging and shaking the lower limb.

4. Course of Treatment: Once a day, 10 days for one course with an interval of 5-7 days between two courses.

Chapter Sixteen
Acute Infective Polyneuroradiculitis

The disease is a special kind of polyneuritis. In general, it belongs to Wei Zheng (Wei Syndrome) in traditional Chinese medicine.

I. ETIOLOGY AND PATHOGENESIS

Accumulation of toxic heat due to invasion by pathogenic wind-heat consumes blood and body fluid, deprives the tendons and muscles of nourishment, giving rise to flaccidity of the limbs.

II. MAIN POINTS OF DIAGNOSIS

1. The patient usually has infection of upper respiratory tract or diarrhea 2-3 weeks prior to the onset of the disease.

2. The disease occurs abruptly with numbness sensation of the limbs. Examination may suggest no significant symptoms. The patient may have hypoesthesia, anesthesia or hyperesthesia at the distal end of the limbs.

3. Myasthenia of the limbs and trunk is the main symptom which will lead to symmetrical paralysis of the limbs and reach its climax within one week. The proximal part of the limbs is worse than the distal part. In severe case, there may be dyspnea.

4. Hypomyotonia, tendon hyporefexia and significant muscular tenderness

of the limbs may occur.

5. Laboratory examination of the cerebrospinal fluid will find that the count of lymphocytes is normal or slightly higherwhile the protein content is significantly increased.

III. DIFFERENTIATION AND
TREATMENT OF COMMON SYNDROMES

1. Excessive Accumulation of Toxic Heat and Retardation of Blood Circulation.

Main Symptoms and Signs: Sudden occurrence of numbness of the limbs, accompanied with fever, thirst, yellow urine, dry stool, red tongue with yellow coating, and rapid pulse.

Therapeutic Principles: Clearing away toxic heat, activating blood circulation and removing obstruction from the channel.

Recipe: Jie Du Huo Xue Tong Luo Tang, modified.

Radix Isatidis	30 g
Lolium Isatidis	15 g
Radix Sophorae Subprostratae	15 g
Lasiosphaera seu Calvatia	9 g
Radix Platycodi	6 g
Ramulus Cinnamomi	6 g
Radix Salviae Miltiorrhizae	30 g
Radix Paeoniae Rubra	15 g
Radix Angelicae Sinensis	15 g
Radix Achyranthis Bidentatae	12 g
Retinervus Luffae Fructus	18 g
Radix Astragali seu Hedysari	15 g
Radix Glycyrrhizae	9 g

Decoct the above ingredients in water for oral use.

Modification: In case of severe toxic heat, Jie Du Tong Luo Tang should be used with modification:

Rhizoma Polygoni Cuspidati	15 g
Herba Bidentis	15 g
Radix Notoginseng	15 g
Radix Salviae Miltiorrhizae	15 g
Caulis Lonicerae	60 g
Rhizoma Dryopteris	30 g

Decoct the above ingredients in water for oral use.

Modification: In case of severe pain, add Rhizoma Corydalis 15 g and Radix Clematidis 15 g.

For dry mouth, mental restlessness, red tongue and rapid pulse, add Radix Glehniae 30 g, Radix Ophiopogonis 15 g and Radix Trichosanthis 12 g.

2. Deficiency of both Qi and Blood and Malnourishment of Muscles and Tendons.

Main Symptoms and Signs: This syndrome mostly occurs at the convalescent stage with such manifestations as flaccidity of the four limbs, general lassitude, normal or poor appetite, normal bowel movement and micturition, thready and forceless pulse, and thin and white tongue coating.

Therapeutic Principles: Tonifying qi, nourishing blood and activating circulation in the channels and collaterals.

Recipe 1: Modified Bu Qi Yang Xue Chu Wei Tang

Radix Astragali seu Hedysari	60 g
Radix Ginseng	10 g
Rhizoma Polygonati	12 g
Radix Codonopsis Pilosulae	15 g
Ramulus Cinnamomi	6 g
Fructus Hordei Germinatus, stir-fried	18 g
Radix Angelicae Sinensis	12 g
Radix Salviae Miltiorrhizae	18 g
Radix Achyranthis Bidentatae 15 g	
Radix Ophiopogonis	15 g
Radix Dipsaci	12 g
Rhizoma Cimicifugae	6 g

Rhizoma Homalomenae	15 g
Herba Cistanchis	15 g
Caulis Spatholobi	18 g

Decoct the above ingredients in water for oral use, one dose a day.

Recipe 2: Du Huo Ji Sheng Tang (Decoction of Angelicae Pubescentis and Taxilli) with modification.

Radix Angelicae Pubescentis	6 g
Ramulus Loranthi	12 g
Radix Gentianae Macrophyllae	6 g
Radix Ledebouriellae	6 g
Herba Asari	3 g
Radix Angelicae Sinensis	12 g
Radix Paeoniae Albae	12 g
Rhizoma Ligustici Chuanxiong	10 g
Radix Rehmanniae Praeparata	12 g
Cortex Eucommiae	9 g
Radix Achyranthis Bidentatae	9 g
Radix Ginseng Rubra	6 g

Decoct the above ingredients in water for oral use.

Acupuncture and Point-injection Therapy: When acupuncture is applied, points Shousanli(LI10) and Hegu(LI4) are taken as the main points, and Jianyu (LI15), Jianliao(SJ14) and Quchi(LI11) as the secondary for the upper limbs; points Shenshu(BL23), Dachangshu(BL25) and Huantiao(GB30) are taken as the main ones, and Zusanli(ST36) and Yanglingquan(GB34) as the secondary for lower limbs. Treatment should be given once every other day and ten times of treatment consisted of one course. Warm needling may obtain even better therapeutic effect.

In point-injection therapy, vitamin B1, Vitamin B12 or Injection of Radix Angelicae Sinensis should be used for the corresponding point injection, 2 ml each point and once a day.

Chapter Seventeen
Epilepsy

Epilepsy is defined as paroxysmal and temporary disturbance of brain characterized by loss of consciousness and muscle tic, abnormal sensation, emotion and behavior. In traditional Chinese medicine, this disease is categorized as "Xian Zheng" (epilepsy syndrome) and "Dian Xian" (epilepsy).

I. ETIOLOGY AND PATHOGENESIS

Epilepsy may have many causes. It is often associated with phlegm. As the saying goes: "No epilepsy develops without phlegm."

1. Congenital Factors. Disturbance of qi and blood of a mother caused by great terror may affect her fetus who may develop epilepsy after birth. Besides, congenital insufficiency of liver-yin and kidney-yin, imbalance of water and fire, impairment of heart and liver are all responsible for disturbance of liver-qi, for mental derangement, convulsion and loss of consciousness. The acquired epilepsy of infants due to frightening is also associated with congenital factors. All that are induced by terror are called convulsive diseases.

2. Blockage of Phlegm in Orifices. There is usually excessive phlegm in infants due to retention of dampness caused by hypofunction of the spleen. Besides, retention of wind and phlegm may still stay in the body after chronic or acute infantile convulsion. It is the accumulation of phlegm in the interior when precipitated by wind, cold or terror, that attacks the upper orifices, therefore inducing epilepsy.

3. Retention of Food in the Middle-Jiao. Improper feeding, or excessive

greasy and sweet foods may all be responsible for the impariment of the spleen and stomach. The dsiorder of receiptive and digestive functions, thus developing infantile dyspepsia. A prolonged retention may transform pathogenic heat, consuming body fluid to from phlegm. Stagnation of phlegm in the middle-jiao makes spleen-qi fails to ascend and stomach-qi to descend.

4. Blood Stasis in the Heart. Accumulation of blood stasis in the heart may be caused by events of birth injury, terror, trauma, or head injury, which may lead mental confusion into epilepsy.

II. MAIN POINTS OF DIAGNOSIS

1. The histories of family, epileptic attack and encephalopathia should be inquired carefully.

2. Clinical manifestations of the disease vary greatly. There may be grand mal, petit mal, rolandic mal and infantile spasms. The grand mal is cahracterized by sudden loss of consciousness, general totanic spasm with apnea, cyanosis and foam in the mouth, which usually last for 1-5 minutes. The patients may then fall into sleep and become conscious a few hours later. The petit mal is characterized by sudden, short loss of consciousness without aurae and muscle tic, accompanied with interruptions of speech and action which usually persisrt for 2- 10 seconds. The patient usually comes to consciousness rapidly.

3. Electroencephalogram examination and tomography may be useful for the diagnosis of epilepsy.

III. DIFFERENTIATION AND TREATMENT
OF COMMON SYNDROMES

Epilepsy can be related to a specific provocation, these include terror, improper diet, accumulation of phlegm and blood stasis. Generally, the syndrome of asthenia accompanied by sthenia is often seen in the infantile convulsion. By sthenia we usually mean phlegm, improper diet and blood stasis. The severity of the disease, the duration of the seizure, the length of the interval are closely related to the depth of the retention of phlegm and the resistance of the body. Initially, retention of phlegm is not deep owing to the exuberance of the vital-qi. The fit is short-lived and the interval is long. With a prolonged process of illness, the vital-qi will be impaired, the retention of phlegm will be deeper, and the seizure will become longer and the interval shorter. If vital-qi fails to prevail pathogenic factors, phlegm will be able to invade the heart, there will appear serious symptoms such as prolonged unconsciousness or coma, or convulsion.

1. Epilepsy Induced by Terror

Main Symptoms and Signs: Sudden panic resulting in confusion and loss of sef-control, sometimes fright and sometimes alarm and restlessness, crying with fear during sleep, tendency to remain in the mother's arms, alternative flush and pallow on the face, red tongue with white fur, taut and rapid or taut and slippery pulse.

Therapeutic Principles: Tranquilizing the mind and resolving phlegm to arrest epilepsy.

Recipe: Modified Polygala Bolus.

Radix Polygala	9 g
Radix Codonopsis Pilosulae	15 g
Poria	9 g
Rhizoma Acori Graminei	9 g
Dens Draconis (To be decocted prior to others)	15 g
Radix Curcumae	9 g
Arisaema cum Bile	9 g
Semen Ziziphi Spinosae	15 g
Semen Biotae	9 g
Periostracum Cicadae	9 g
Radix Asparagi	9 g

All the above drugs are to be decocted in water for oral administration.

2. Epilepsy due to Accumulation of Phlegm

Main Symptoms and Signs: Convulsion of extremities during a fit of epilepsy, unconsciousness or vertigo, headache and abdominal pain, accompanied with stridor produced by phlegm in the throat, salivation, yellow face, thick fur of the tongue, and slippery and rapid pulse.

Therapeutic Principles: Removing phlegm and inducing resuscitation.

Recipe: Modified Phlegm-removing Decoction.

Rhizoma Pinelliae	6 g
Pericarpium Citri Reticulatae	6 g
Poria	9 g
Caulis Bambusae in taenis	6 g
Fructus Aurantii	9 g
Rhizoma Gastrodiae	9 g
Arisaema cum Bile	9 g
Rhizoma Acori Graminei	9 g
Scorpio	6 g
Radix Glycyrrhizae	3 g

All the above drugs are to be decocted in water for oral administration.

3. Epilepsy due to Blood Stasis

Main Symptoms and Signs: With a history of birth injury or trauma often manifested as paroxysmal localized headache, occasional vomiting, paroxysmal convulsion of the whole body or half body or local region upon attack, dark purple tongue with ecchymoses, thready and unsmooth pulse and dark purple superficial venule of the index finger.

Therapeutic Principles: Promoting blood circulation to remove blood stasis, waking up the patient from unconsciousness and arresting epilepsy.

Recipe: Modified Decoction for Activating Blood Circulation.

Rhizoma Ligustici Chuanxiong	6 g
Radix Paeoniae Rubra	9 g
Semen Persicae	9 g
Flos Carthami	9 g
Bulbus et Radix Allii Fistulosi	3 pieces
Rhizoma Zingiberis	9 g
Fructus Ziziphi Jujubae	7 pieces

Radix Salviae Miltiorrhizae 12 g

Moschus (Grind into powder to be taken after being infused in the finished decoction) 1.5 g

All the above drugs except musk are to be decocted in water for oral administration.

In case of deficiency of qi, add 30 grams of astragalus root (Radix Astragali seu Hedysari) and 12 grams of dangshen (Radix Codonopsis Pilosulae) into the above mentioned recipe.

4. Epilepsy due to Improper Diet

Main Symptoms and Signs: This type of epilepsy is characterized, among others, by abdominal flatulence, acid vomitus, foul-smelling stools, and thick greasy fur on the tongue.

Therapeutic Principles: Relieving dyspepsia and resolving phlegm; calming endopathogenic wind.

Recipe: Baohe Wan (Lenitive Pill), modified.

Fructus Crataegi Praeparata	12 g
Massa Fermentata Medicinalis	9 g
Semen Arecae	9 g
Fructus Forsythiae	9 g
Flos Chrysanthemi	9 g
Ramulus Uncariae cum Uncis	9 g
Rhizoma Pinelliae	6 g
Fructus Aurantii Immaturus	6 g

All the above drugs are to be decocted in water for oral administration.

Modification: Constipation can be combated by adding Radix et Rhizoma Rhei (Decocted later).

5. Epilepsy due to Blood Stasis in Children

Main Symptoms and Signs: This type of epilepsy often occurs in the child with previous trauma or birth injury. The epileptic child usually has a headache in a fixed position and vomiting in severe case. The tongue proper is deep purplish with ecchymoses on it.

Therapeutic Principles: Promoting blood circulation by removing blood stasis.

Recipe: Tongqiao Huoxue Tang (Decoction for Activating Blood Circulation), modified.

Rhizoma Ligustici	6 g
Radix Paeoniae Rubra	9 g
Semen Persicae	9 g
Flos Carthami	9 g
Allium Fistulosum	3 segments
Radix Salvae Miltiorrhizae	12 g
Fructus Ziziphi Jujubae	5
Moschus (Powdered and mixed with the decoction)	0.15 g

All the above drugs are to be decocted in water for oral administration.

Modification: Deficiency of liver-yin and kidney-yin due to prolonged and recurrent epilepsy can be combated by using modified Zuogui Wan to replenish essence and tonify the kidney. Deficiency of qi and blood in the heart and spleen can be treated by using Guipi Wan (modified) to invigorate the heart and spleen.

IV. OTHER THERAPIES

Recipe: Modified Baijin Wan

Fructus Canarii	3 g
Alumen	3 g
Magnetitum	18 g
Radix Polygalae	9 g
Radix Curcumae	9 g
Rhizoma Acori Graminei	9 g
Radix Ophiopogonis	9 g
Cinnabaris	3 g

Direction: All the ingredients above are mixed and powdered, 1.5 g is taken eache time, three times daily. This method is claimed to be effective against epilepsy due to terror or phlegm.

V. PREVENTION AND NURSING

1. The pregnant woman should keep physically and mentally healthy. Birth injurs should be avoided.

2. Infants with a history of febrile seizures should be given antipyretic and anticonfulsant.

3. Infantile dyspepsia can be combated by regular feeding.

4. The epileptic child should not be allowed to move about himself. During the onset of fits, the respiratory tract should be kept unobstructed to avoid asphyxia. Emergent treatment should be taken at once.

Chapter Eighteen
Infantile Paralysis

Infantile paralysis, which is called poliomyelitis in modern medicine, belongs to epidemic febrile disease. It is also called "flaccid paralysis in leg muscles". At the preparalytic stage, the manifestations are fever, cough, congestion of throat, vomiting, diarrhea and muscular pain (limbache), and then limb weakness and muscle relaxation. At the postparalytic stage, muscular atrophy and skeleton deformity are the first evidence in clinical features.

Infantile paralysis tends to occur in summer and autumn, mostly attacking the young children of 1-5 years of age. In mild cases the patient could recover his health thoroughly, but in the severe cases, the patient may develop severe paralysis called sequels. The patient may acquire lifelong immunity after an attack.

I. ETIOLOGY AND PATHOGENESIS

Seasonal epidemic pathogens such as wind, dampness and heat invade the lung and stomach channels through mouth and nose, thus, at the beginning of the disease, it is mostly manifested by the syndrome of the invasion of pathogens in the lung and stomach, such as fever, cough, congestion of throat, or vomiting and diarrhea. Then the pathogens flow into the channels and collaterals, and deranges qi and blood systems, thus manifestations such as muscular pain will appear.

The lung controls qi and converges all the vessels of the body. The stomach is the sea of water and food, and the source of transformation of qi and blood, nourishing of urogenital region of the body, promoting muscles and tendons, and relieving rigidity of joints. If the lung and stomach are steamed by the dampness and heat, the transformed fire will consume the body fluid, resulting in lack of fluid in the lung and kidney. So the liver is not nourished. In later stage, the syndrome of flaccidity of muscles and bones would occur.

II. MAIN POINTS OF DIAGNOSIS

1. The disease occurse mostly in summer and autumn months.

2. The manifestations are fever, headache, sore throat, nausea and muscular pain of the whole body. The fever may be double peaked. After the second fever, the muscle pain, tenderness and paralysis would occur. Actually, the fever also could be single peaked, or the parlysis could directly occur.

3. the syndrome of invasion of the lung and stomach by pathogenic factors presents similar symptoms and signs, to the common cold usually lasts for about one week, and fevr does not occur again once it subsides. If double quotidian fever and pain in the limbs and trunk are present, the possibility of this disease is great.

4. The paralysis is characterized by flaccidity and asymmetry. Paralysis of lower limbs is more frequent than that of the upper ones. Paralysis of proximal muscles is more severe than that of distal muscles. Tendon reflex disappears, with abdominal muscles, intercostal muscles and diaphragms involved. Sensation may be nonspecific.

5. The laboraory examination usually reveals elevation of the cells of CSF, but seldom above the number of 500, among which the lymphocytes constitute the most of the number of cells. When cells reduce after 2-3 weeks, on the contrary, the protein may gradually elevate, marked by cell-protein dissociation.

III. DIFFERENTIATION AND
TREATMENT OF COMMON SYNDROMES

1. Stagnation of Pathogenic Factors in the Lung and Stomach (Prodromal

Stage)

Main Symptoms and Signs: Fever, sweating, cough, running nose, congestion of throat and sore-throat, accompanied by vomiting, diarrhea or abdominal pain, lethargy or irritability, red tongue with greasy fur.

This syndrome occurs at the early stage when the lung and stomach are diseased at the same time. Invasion of the lung by pathogenic factor impairs its function in descending, and thereby results in fever, cough, runny nose and inflamed throat. Retention of damp-heat in the spleen and stomach impairs their function in ascending and descending with the result of vomiting and loose stools, a red tongue with thin and sticky coating and a rapid pulse are both signs of wind, damp and heat.

Therapeutic Principles: Dispelling wind and relieving exterior syndrome; clearing away heat and promoting diuresis.

Recipe: Gegen Qinlian Tang (Decoction of Radix Puerariae, Radix Scutellariae and Rhizoma Coptidis) and Ganlu Xiaodu Dan, modified.

Radix Puerariae	9 g
Radix Scutellariae	6 g
Herba Agastachis	9 g
Herba Artemisiae Scopariae	18 g
Poria	9 g
Fructus Forsythiae	9 g
Rhizoma Acori Graminei	9 g
Radix Isatidis	12 g
Radix Platycodi	6 g

All the above drugs are to be decocted in water for oral administration.

Modification: In case of severe damp pathogens, greasy fur, Semen Coicis 12 g, Cortex Magnoliae Officinalis 9 g and Rhizoma Pinelliae 6 g should be added. In case of constipation, Fructus Trichosanthis (12 g) should be added.

2. Invasion of Pathogenic Factors into Channels and Collaterals (Preparalytic Stage)

Main Symptoms and Signs: Second fever, muscle pain, difficulty in turning over, refusal to be touched or held in arms, irritability or lethargy, and then development of paralysis; red tongue with greasy fur.

When pathogenic facotrs are transmitted inward, heat disappears but damp remains. Damp then turns into heat, and thereby gives rise to retention of damp-heat in the interior. Thise explains recurrence of fever and profuse sweating. Invasion of the channels and collaterals by damp-heat causes derangement of qi, which is the cause of pain in the limbs and trunk, reluctance to be patted and held, and reslessness with crying. A red tongue with thin, sticky and slightly yellow coating, and a weak-floating and rapid pulse are signs of damp-heat.

Therapeutic Principles: Dispelling heat and resolving dampment of paralysis; relieving rigidity of muscles and activating collaterals.

Recipe: Sanmiao Wan (Pill of Three Ingredients with Wonderful Effects) and Qingluo Yin , modified.

Rhizoma Atractylodis Praeparatae	9 g
Radix Achyranthis Bidentatae	9 g
Radix gentianae Macrophyllae	9 g
Radix Puerariae	9 g
Semen Coicis	12 g
Caulis Trachelospermi	12 g
Cortex Phellodendri	6 g
Radix Paeoniae Rubra	9 g
Radix Angelicae Sinensis	9 g
Radix Salviae Miltiorrhizae	9 g
Flos Lonicerae Vine	30 g

All the above drugs are to be decocted in water for oral administration.

Modification: For patient with facial hemiparalysis due to abundant wind and phlegm pathogens, Rhizoma Typhonii 9g, Bombyx Batryticatus 9 g, and Scorpio 6 g should be added. For patient with severe dampness, Herba Artemisiae Scopariae 15 g should be added.

3. Qi Deficiency and Blood Stasis (Paralysis Phase Restoration Stage)

Main Symptoms and Signs: Following fever, paralysis and extreme weakness, or squint of mouth and eyes would occur. The fur on the tongue is pale and thin.

This syndrome manifest as disappearance of pathogenic factors and deficiency of body resistance. Deficiency of qi with stagnation of blood deprives the tendons and muscles of nourishment, and thereby results in weakness and paralysis of the limbs and trunk. Deficiency of qi and blood in a prolonged case leads to pale complexion. A pale tongue with thin coating, and a thready and weak pulse are both signs of deficiency of qi and blood.

Therapeutic Principles: Nourishing the blood by invigorating qi; promoting blood circulation to remove obstruction in the channels.

Recipe: Buyang Huanwu Tang (Decoction for Treating Paralysis)

Radix Astragali seu Hedysari	15 g
Caulis Spatholobi	15 g
Radix Angelicae Sinensis	9 g
Rhizoma Ligustici Chuanxiong	6 g
Semen Persicae	6 g
Lumbricus	6 g
Radix Paeoniae Rubra	9 g
Ramulus Mori	9 g
Fructus Liquidambairs	9 g
Radix Glycyrrhizae	3 g

All the above drugs are to be decocted in water for oral administration.

Modification: In case of paralysis of upper limbs, Ramulus Cinnamomi 9 g should be added. In case of paralysis of lower limbs, Cortex Eucommiae 9 g, Radix Achyranthis Bidentatae 9 g, Ramulus Lorathi 9 g should be added. In case of thirst and red tongue, Rhizoma Anemarrhenae 9 g, Radix Ophiopogonis 9 g should be added.

4. Deficiency of Liver-Yin and Kidney-Yin (Sequal Stage)

Main Symptoms and Signs: Long time of paralysis, muscle atrophy and low skin temperature, failure of the extremities to move back to the original deformed limbs, pale tongue without fur.

Therapeutic Principles: Tonifying the liver and kidney, promoting the flow of qi by warming the channels.

Recipe: Yougui Wan (The Kidney-yang-reinforcing Bolus), modified.

Rhizoma Rehmanniae Praeparata	12 g
Rhizoma Dioscoreae	12 g
Fructus Corni	12 g

Semen Cruscutae	12 g
Cortex Eucommiae	9 g
Fructus Lycii	9 g
Colla Cornu Cervi	9 g
Radix Angelicae Sinensis	9 g
Lumbricus	9 g
Radix Aconiti	6 g
Cortex Cinnamomi	6 g
Caulis Spatholobi	15 g

All the above drugs are to be decocted in water for oral administration.

Modification: In case of smooth and red tongue without fur, hectic fever, Radix Aconiti and Cortex Cinnamomi should be replaced by Rhizoma Anemarrhenae 6 g and Radix Ophiopogonis 15 g, Additional Huqian Wan may be taken, 3-6 g a time, twice to three times daily.

OTHER THERAPIES

1. Cooked spinal cord of a pig or an ox and some soybean, suitable in paralysis and squel stage.

2. Acupuncture treatment of paralysis.

1) Upper limbs: Jiaji(EX-B2), Jianyu(LI15), Jianzhen(SI15), Quchi(LI11), Waiguan(SJ5), Hegu(LI4).

2) Lower limbs: Huantiao(GB30), Yinlingquan(SP9), Kunlun(BL60), Taixi(KI3), Shenshu(BL23), Yaoyangguan(DU3). In case of eversion, needle points at the medial aspect of the leg such as Sanyinjiao(SP6) and Shangqiu (SP5). In case of inversion, needle points at the lateral aspect of the leg such as Xuanzhong(GB39) and Qiuxu(GB40).

3) Facial nerve: Jiache(ST6), Dicang(ST4), Hegu(LI4).

4) Diaphragm: Geshu(BL17), Qimen(LR14), Jiuwei(RN15).

5) Abdominal muscle: Zhongwan(RN12), Tianshu(ST25), Qihai(RN6).

6) Sphincter vesicae: Shenshu(BL23), Pangguangshu(BL28), Zhongji

(RN30), Guanyuan(RN4), Yinlingquan(SP9).

All the above drugs are to be decocted in water for oral administration.

When the disease develops to paralysis, application of acupuncture is conductive to the recovery, and also reduces the incidence of after-effects. Some sick children with more than one year's duration of disease can still expect improvement with the help of acupuncture.

PREVENTION AND NURSING

1. In the epidemic period, avoid overworking and catching cold. Postponereceiving vaccines and undergoing unnecessary operation, in order to prevent development from abortive type to paralysis type.

2. The ill children should be isolated for 40 days from the day of onset. Stools should be disinfected, clothes exposed in the sun.

3. The young children of 2-7 months should take OPV (oral poliovirus vaccine). The immunization is reliable without general side effect or local side effect such as the adverse reaction seen in the stomach and intestines.

4. The sick children should be kept in bed. The wet hot compress is used for releasing the muscle pain. If paralysis occurs, the limbs should be put in the functional positions to prevent from deformed descendent limbs.

Chapter Nineteen
Senile Dementia

Senile dementia denotes the occurrence of aphrenia in the old age or the pre-senile period. This affection includes three major kinds: senile dementia (amounting to 50% and more), cerebrovascular dementia and dementia induced by many other disorders. Senile dementia is often seen in clinical practice. In traditional Chinese medicine, this affection is ascribed to the categories of "dullness", "amnesia", "general debility", "depression syndrome", "insanity and maniac" etc.. According to the symptom-sign differentiation of traditional Chinese medicine, this affection can be classified into two types: the deficiency type and the excess type. The former includes patterns of insufficiency of sea of marrow, deficiency of kidney and liver; the latter includes patterns of abundant fire in heart and deficiency of both spleen and kidney, phlegm turbidity in yang orifices, qi stagnancy and blood stasis.

I. DIFFERENTIATION AND TREATMENT OF COMMON SYNDROMES

1. Type of Heart Disorder

Main Symptoms and Signs: Palpitation, liability to start, failure to concentrate attention, fatigue, insomnia, dreaminess.

Recipe:

Radix Asparagi	10 g
Radix Ophiopogonis	10 g
Radix Rehmanniae	10 g
Bulbus Lilli	10 g
Radix Codonopsis Pilosulae	10 g
Radix Astragali seu hedysari	10 g

| Rhizoma Atractylodis | 10 g |
| Macrocephalae | 10 g |

2. Type of Liver Yang

Main Symptoms and Signs: Headache, distention of head, dizziness, irritability, tinnitus, constipation, red urine, rapid and forceful pulse.

Recipe:

Concha Haliotidis	30 g
Magnetitum	30 g
Os Draconis	25 g
Rhizoma Ligustici Chuanxiong	15 g
Ramulus Uncariae cum Uncis	10 g
Rhizoma Ligustici	10 g

3. Type of Qi Depression

Main Symptoms and Signs: Liability to upset, sigh, suffocation, poor appetite, distention of flanks, bitter mouth.

Recipe:

Radix Bupleuri	10 g
Rhizoma Cyperi	10 g
Radix Aucklandiae	10 g
Fructus Aurantii Immaturus	10 g
Radix Linderae	10 g
Pericarpium Citri Reticulatae Viride	6 g
Radix Curcumae	15 g

4. Type of Yin Deficiency

Main Symptoms and Signs: Bitter mouth, dry throat, tinnitus, sweating, rapid slender pulse.

Recipe:

Herba Dendrobii	20 g
Radix Rehmanniae	15 g
Radix Ophiopogonis	15 g
Radix Scrophulariae	10 g
Fructus Mume	10 g
Fructus Schisandrae	10 g

5. Type of Yang Deficiency

Main Symptoms and Signs: Aversion to cold, lustreless complexion, sore waist and weak feet, poor appetite, slender and forceless pulse.

Recipe:

Radix Aconiti Praeparata	10 g
Rhizoma Zingiberis	10 g
Cortex Cinnamomi	5 g
Radix Glycyrrhizae	5 g
Herba Cistanchis	15 g
Radix Morindae Officinalis	15 g

6. Type of Inevident Manifestations

Recipe:

Rhizoma Zedoariae	10 g
Radix et Rhizoma Rhei	10 g
Radix Paeoniae Rubra	15 g

Thirty patients were treated with the above mentioned method for six months. Of whom, 7 gained marked improvement and 16 improved.

II. SIMPLE RECIPES AND PROVED RECIPES

1. Coptidis Antidotal Decoction

Recipe:

Rhizoma Coptidis	9 g
Radix Scutellariae	9 g
Cortex Phellodendri	9 g
Fructus Gardeniae	9 g

All the above drugs are to be decocted in water for oral administration. One dose a day to be taken in two separate portions. One course of treatment consisting of three months.

The above method was used in treatment of 24 cases, of whom, the improvement rate for dyskinesia amounted to 66%, that for sensory disturbance amounted to 55%, that for emotional disturbance amounted to 13%, that for sleep disturbance amounted to 88%, that for repression syndrome amounted to 72%, that for decrease of intelligence amounted to 80%. As compared with the controls given synthetic drugs, the improvement rate was higher in the group given herbal drugs.

2. Anti-encephalatrophy Decoction

Recipe:

Radix Astragali seu Hedysari	60 g
Radix Rehmanniae	30 g
Poria	30 g
Radix Polygoni Multiflori	15 g
Concretio Silicea Bambusae	15 g
Radix Angelicae Sinensis	10 g
Rhizoma Ligustici Chuanxiong	10 g
Lumbricus	10 g
Radix Ophiopogonis	10 g
Fructus Schisandrae	10 g
Rhizoma Acori Graminei	10 g
Squama Manitis	10 g
Radix Angelicae Dahuricae	10 g
Rhizoma Arisaematis	10 g

Modifications: In case of qi deficiency as a main factor, Radix Ginseng 5 g, Radix Codonopsis Pilosulae 10 g were added; Caulis Spatholobi added for blood deficiency; Herba Lonicerae 10 g and Hirudo 5 g added for blood stasis (Infusion of Hirudo P owder is of better effect for hyperlipodemia of high blood viscosity.); Radix Notoginseng 3 g added for blood stasis with hemorrhage; Flos Sophorae or Flos Sophorae Immaturus 10 g added for blood heat with hemorrhage; Radix Astragali seu Hedysari, adix Polygoni Multiflori, Radix Angelicae Dahuricae reduced and Fructus Ligustri Lucidi 10 g, Fructus Corni 10 g added for simple deficiency of yin elements; Radix Aconiti Praeparata 10 g, Cortex Cinnamomi 5 g, Herba Cistanchis 10 g, Radix Morindae Officinalis 10 g added for yang deficiency; Oltheca Mantidis added for incontinence of urine; Rhizoma Atractylodis Macrocephalae added for salivation; Scolopendra 10 g, Ramulus Uncariae cum

Uncis 10 g added for dysbasia; medicinal leaven 10 g added for anorexia; Ramulus Cinnamomi 10 g added for lassitude of the upper limbs; Ramulus Mori 10 g added for lassitude of the lower limbs; Radix Astragali seu Hedysari, Radix Polygoni Multiflori, Radix Angelicae Dahuricae substracted and Arisaemae cum Bile 10 g, Spica Prunellae 10 g and Succus Bambusae 1 amp added for sthenic phlegm; Semen Biotae 10 g added for amnesia; Poria cum Ligno Hospite 10 g, Semen Ziziphi Jujubae 10 g, Dens Draconis 30 g added for listlessness, insomnia and deafness.

All the above drugs are to be decocted in water for oral administration. To be taken one dose daily in two separate portions. One course of treatment consisting of one month.

8 cases were treated with the above method, one of them was cured and six cases gained effectiveness.

3. Tonifying Kidney and Benefiting Brain Decoction

    Recipe:

Radix Astragali seu Hedysari	15 g
Radix Codonopsis Pilosulae	15 g
Radix Polygoni Multiflori	15 g
Fructus Lycii	15 g
Arillus Longan	15 g
Rhizoma Dioscoreae	15 g
Radix Angelicae Sinensis	15 g
Rhizoma Acori Graminei	10 g
Radix Polygalae	10 g
Fructus Alpiniae Oxyphyllae	10 g
Radix Morindae Officinalis	10 g
Fructus Corni	10 g
Semen Cuscutae	10 g
Rhizoma Gastrodiae	10 g
Rhizoma Rehmanniae	20 g
Concha Margaritifera Usta	30 g

Modifications: In case of poor appetite, abdominal dsitention and loose stool, the dosage of Radix Astragali seu Hedysari and Radix Codonopsis Pilosulae should be added to 30-40 g respectively, Rhizoma Atractylodis Macrocephallae 10 g, Poria 10 g, Herba Agastachis 10 g and Herba Eupatorii 10 g be added; Coptidis Antidortal Decoction could be used for dysphoria and insomnia, dry stool and dark urine; Radix Salviae Miltiorrhizae 10 g, Radix Paeoniae Rubra 10 g, Rhizoma Ligustici Chuanxiong 10g added for incoherent speech, repeat relapse of lingering illness, dark tongue proper with ecchymoses. Besides, Adding rabbit's brain and pig's spinal marrow into the decoction might yield good effect.

All the above drugs are to be decocted in water for oral administration. One course of treatment consisting of at least 30 days.

Twenty-five patients were treated with the above method. The course of treatment ranged from 60 to 180 days.

Result: 8 got marked effect, 10 got effectiveness. The therapeutic effect in patients of mild and moderate condition was better than that in those of severe condition. The longer the medication period, the better the effect. Marked improvement was seen in speech, memory and movement, changes were not obvious in ability of judgement and thinking.

4. Lightening Body Decoction

Recipe:

Herba Artemisiae Scopariae	40 g
Radix Polygoni Multiflori	20 g
Radix Puerariae	20 g
Fructus Rosae Laevigatae	30 g
Rhizoma Arismatis	15 g
Radix et Rhizoma Rhei	10 g
Pulvis Notoginseng	5 g

All the above drugs are to be decocted in water for oral administration. One course of treatment consisting of 5-7 days. In general four courses were necessary.

32 cases were treated with this method, 9 got marked effect, 18 got response with a total effective rate of 84.4%. The effective rate in the age group of 50 to 59 years accounted for 91.6%, but that in the age group of 70 and odd years was only 66.7%.

5. Restoring Juvenescence Decoction

Recipe:

Fructus Corni	20 g
Poria	20 g
Cortex Eucommiae	20 g
Rhizoma Dioscoreae	30 g
Fructus Lycii	30 g
Rhizoma Acori Graminei	30 g
Radix Rehmanniae	15 g
Radix Achyranthis Bidentatae	15 g
Herba Cistanchis	15 g
Fructus Schisandrae	15 g
Fructus Ziziphi Jujubae	15 g
Fructus Broussonetiae Papyriferae	10 g
Fructus Foeniculi	10 g
Radix Polygalae	10 g
Rhizoma Zingiberis	6 g

All the above drugs are to be decocted in water for oral administration. One course of treatment consisting of three weeks.

14 cases were treated with the above method and 5 of them were cured, 4 got marked effect, 3 improved. 12 cases were examined again by CT, of which 1 case had its focus disappeared, 3 had their foci reduced and 7 had no change, 1 case had its focus expanded.

6. Opening Orifices and Activating Blood Decoction

Recipe:

Radix Paeoniae Rubra	12 g
Rhizoma Ligustici Chuanxiong	6 g
Radix Angelicae Sinensis	12 g
Semen Persicae	10 g
Flos Carthami	10 g
Moschus	0.2 g
Rhizoma Acori Graminei	12 g
Radix Astragali seu Hedysari	30 g
Fructus Lycii	15 g

Fructus Crataegi	15 g
Fructus Ziziphi Jujubae	510 g
Rhizoma Zingiberis	3 g

Modifications: In case of dizziness and headache, Rhizoma Gastrodiae 10 g, Spica Prunellae 10 g were added; Periostracum Cicadae 5 g, Rhizoma Rehmanniae 10 g added for tinnitus and deafness; Fructus Liquidambaris 10 g and Semen Oroxyli 10 g added for jumbled speech; Semen Jujubae 10 g, Radix Salviae Miltiorrhizae 10 g and Succinum 5 g added for insomnia and amnesia; Flos Chrysanthemi 10 g, Carapax Trionycis 10 g and Fructus Gardeniae 10g added for dysphoria and irritability; Fructus Polygoni Multiflori Praeparata 10 g, Rhizoma Rehmanniae 10 g added for complication of yin deficiency; Fructus Aurantii 10 g and Radix Aucklandiae 10 g added for qi stagnancey; Caulis Bambusae in Taeniam 5 g and Radix Polygalae 10 g added for complication of phlegm-turbidity.

The above method was used in treating 7 dementia cases, 5 got marked effect and 2 got effectiveness. Response was seen after medication of half of a month. The effect increased along with the lengthening of treating time. It was found in examinations that the blood flow in brain improved markedly, which was not in positive proportion with the result seen in CT.

7. Decoction for Removing Blood Stasis from Blood Chamber Associated with Reducing Phlegm Method

Recipe:

Semen Persicae	12 g
Flos Carthami	9 g
Radix Angelicae Sinensis	9 g
Radix Rehmanniae	9 g
Radix Achyranthis Bidentatae	9 g
Radix Paeoniae Rubra	6 g
Fructus Aurantii	6 g
Rhizoma Ligustici Chuanxiong	5 g
Radix Platycodi	5 g
Radix Glycyrrhizae	3 g
Radix Bupleuri	3 g

Modifications: In case of blocade of phlegm-turrbidity in the interior, Pericarpium Citri Reticulatae 5 g, Rhizoma Pinelliae 10 g, Poria 10 g, Rhizoma Alismatis 10 g, Semen Plantaginis 10 g are added; Radix Scutellariae 10 g, Rhizoma Coptidis 3 g added for depressive phlegm turning into fire; Radix Polygalae 10 g, Radix Curcumae 10 g, Rhizoma Acori Graminei 10 g, Rhizoma Pinelliae 10 g and Poria 10 g, Pericarpium Citri Reticulatae 6 g added for mental depression, indifferent expression, dull intelligence and incoherent speech; Concretio Silicea Bambusae 10 g, Bombyx Batryticatus 10 g, Radix Codonopsis Pilosulae 10 g, Radix Asttragali seu Hedysari 10 g, Radix Polygalae 10 g, Semen Biotae 10 g, Semen Ziziphi Jujubae 10 g added for trance, palpitation, fatigue of limbs, poor appetite, light tongue proper, slender forceless pulse; 10 g of Chlorite Pills for Expelling Phlegm (wraped with a piece of gauze and decocted in water) added for impatience, headache, insomnia, flushing face, red eyes, crimson tongue proper, big slippery rapid and taut pulse; Radix Ophiopogonis 10 g, Bulbus Fritillariae Thunbergii 10 g, Poria Ligno Hospite 10 g added for liability to fear, bony constitution, flushing face, red tongue proper, slender and rapid pulse.

All the above drugs are to be decocted in water for oral administration. One course of treatment consisting of two weeks.

The above method was used in treating 40 dementia cases. After three treating courses, 29 cases were cured and 15 cases improved, with a total effective rate of 97.5%. Besides, a control group of 40 cases was given NA inositolipid 0. 2 g, gama- aminobutyric acid 0.5 g, trilafon 2-4 mg or doxepin 25 mg per os t. i. d. If patients were complicated with cerebral angiospasm or cerebral thrombosis, low molecule dextran at 250 ml was instilled intravenously q. d. One course of treatment consisting of two weeks.

Result: 15 cases gained recovery, 11 improved. The effective rate accounted for 65%. to compare the results in the two groups, there was significant difference (P<0.05). According to the follow-up of half a year, there was no flucuation in the treatment group, two cases fluctuated in the control group, so they were given herbal Chinese drugs.

8. The Method of Benefiting Kidney and Activating Blood Circulation

1) For patients of yin-deficiency of kidney

Recipe:

Fructus Corni   15 g

Rhizoma Dioscoreae	15 g
Fructus Lycii	15 g
Herba Ecliptae	15 g
Fructus Ligustri Lucidi	15 g
Radix Polygoni Multiflori Praeparata	15 g
Fructus Psoraleae	15 g
Placenta Hominis	15 g
Radix Alismatis	10 g

2) For patients of yang-deficiency of kidney

Recipe:

Radix Aconiti Praeparata	10 g
Placenta Hominis	15 g
Rhizoma Curculiginis	15 g
Herba Epimedii	15 g
Herba Cistanchis	15 g
Fructus Corni	15 g
Fructus Psoraleae	15 g
Radix Angelicae Sinensis	15 g
Radix Alismatis	15 g
Cortex Cinnamomi	5 g

3) For patients with both deficiency of yin and yang in kidney

Recipe:

Radix Aconiti Praeparata	10 g
Fructus Corni	15 g
Radix Rehmanniae	15 g
Rhizoma Dioscoreae	15 g
Plancenta Hominis	15 g
Radix Polygoni Multiflori Praeparata	15 g
Herba Cistanchis	15 g
Radix Alismatis	15 g

Modification: For evident cold limbs, add the dosage of Radix Aconiti Praeparata to 15 g; Cortex Phellodendri 10 g, Rhizoma Anemarrhenae 10 g for evident yin deficency with sthenic fire; Rhizoma Ligustici Chuanxiong 10 g, Flos

Carthami 10 g, Semen Persicae 10 g, Radix Paeniae Rubra 10 g, Radix Salviae Miltiorrhizae 10 g, Radix Achyranthis Bidentate 10 g added for activating blood circulation and reducing stasis; Radix Polygalae 10 g, Calamus 10 g and Cortex Albiziae 10 g added for wakening brain and opening orifices.

All the above drugs are to be decocted in water for oral administration. A testing course consisting of one month.

18 cases were treated with the above method. After the treatment of three to twelve months, 8 cases were cured and 7 cases gained response.

III. OTHER THERAPIES

1. Acupuncture and Infravenous Instillation
1) Acupuncture
Principal points: Shenting (DU24), Baihui (DU20), Fengchi (GB20), Shenmen(HT7), Dazhong(KI4).

Subordinate points: Taichong(LR3), Taixi(KI3), Zusanli(ST36), Daling (PC7), Sanyinjiao(SP6).

Manipulation: Normal tonification and sedation. Treatment given once a day for one month.

2) Intravenous instillation
500 mg of cytodiphosphocholine was instilled once a day for half a month.

The above methods were used for treating 36 cases being divided randomly into two groups (18 cases each). In the group of acupuncture in combination with drug therapy, 15 cases got marked effect, accounting for 83.3%. In the group of given drug alone, 9 got marked effect, accounting for 50%. This suggested that the effect of combined use of acupuncture and drug was more evident in enhancing intelligence than the effect of drug alone ($P<0.01$). All the 36 cases were of mild and moderate dementia with evident memory disturbance.

2. Acupuncture and Point Injection
1) Acupuncture
Principal points: Baihui (DU20), Qiangjian (DU18), Naohu (DU17),

Shuigou(DU26).

Subordinate points: Shenmen(HT7), Tongli(HT5), Sanyinjiao(SP6).

Modifications: For abnormal blood fat, Neiguan(PC6) should be punctured; Naogan(AT3,4i) brain stem used for unconsciousness; Daling(PC7) punctured for restlessness and wrangle at night; Dicang(ST4) punctured for salivation; Shanglingquan(EX) punctured for dyslalia or difficult swallowing; the III lateral line of the head needling used for incontinence of urination and defecation; Hegu (LI4), Huantiao(GB30) and Zusanli(ST36) stimulated with electroacupuncture for hemiplegia; Yanglingquan(GB34) punctured for strengthlessness of lower limbs while walking.

2) Point injection

Points of group A: Yamen(DU15), Ganshu(BL18), Shenshu(BL23).

Points of group B: Dazhui(DU14), Fengchi(GB20), Zusanli(ST36).

Manipulation: Treatment given once every other day. After acupuncture, point injection was added. When stimulating different points, needles were retained for twenty minutes. When point injection is applied, pints of group A and B are used alternatively. Acetylglutamic acid solutionof 1 ml is injected into each point. Fifteen times of treatment consisted of one course, and results are observed after three courses.

21 cases of cerebrovascular dementia were treated with the above methods. Two of them got marked effect, 7 gained response, 9 improved. The total effective rate accounted for 85.71%.

Chapter Twenty
Meniere's Disease

Meniere's disease is also known as hydrops of memebranous labyrinth. Its clinical characteristics are paroxysmal dizziness, fluctuating deafness, tinnitus and a feeling of fullness in the ear. It belongs to the category of "Xuan Yun" (dizziness) in traditional Chinese medicine.

I. MAIN POINTS OF DIAGNOSIS

1. It occurs most often in middle-aged males, as a result of fatigue, change in mood and lack of sleep.

2. The patient suffers from paroxysmal vertigo and a sensation of rotating around or floating-and-sinking, accompanied with spontaneous nystagemus, nausea, vomiting, pallor and cold sweating. The dizziness may last for several minutes or even several hours, but the patient is conscious.

3. Constant tinnitus occurs, which is aggravated before or after the attack of the disease.

4. The patient has sensorineural deafness. It fluctuates prior to and after the attack of the disease. Hyper-sensitive sign to high-pitch sound may occur.

5. The patient has a feeling of fullness in the ear and head.

6. Examination show the drum membrane is normal. There is horizontal or slightly rotatory nystagmus during the attack. Hearing test indicates a sensorineural hypoacusis and recruitment may be present. The vestibular function

test shows that its function is reduced during the period of the attack.

7. Glycerin test shows positive.

II. DIFFERENTIATION AND
TREATMENT OF COMMON SYNDROMES

1. Hyperactivity of Liver-yang

Main Symptoms and Signs: Vertigo occurs mostly after a change in mood. Tinnitus like chattering sound of machine is present, accompanied with resless-ness, irritability, headache and a feeling of fullness in the ear as well as flushing face, red eyes, a bitter taste in the mouth and driness in the throat. The tongue is red and its fur yellow. The pulse is taut and rapid.

Therapeutic Principle: Calming the liver to stop endogenous wind and nour-ishing yin to suppress yang.

Recipe: Decoction of Gastrodia and Uncaria

Rhizoma Gastrodiae	9 g
Radix Scutellariae	9 g
Radix Achyranthis Bidentatae	9 g
Cortex Eucommiae	9 g
Ramulus Uncariae cum Uncis (decocted later)	15 g
Fructus Gardeniae	15 g
Herba Leonuri	15 g
Ramulus Loranthi	15 g
Caulis Polygoni Multiflori	15 g
Poria cum Ligno Hospite	15 g
Concha Haliotidis	30 g (decocted first)

All the above drugs are to be decocted in water for oral administration.

2. Turbid Phlegm Obstruction in the Middle-jiao

Main Symptoms and Signs: There are such symptoms as dizziness and shakiness, which will be aggravated by movements, accompanied with nausea, vomiting, a sensation of heaviness in the head as if it were tightly wrapped up, a feeling of fullness in the chest and poor appetite. The fur of the tongue is white and greasy and the pulse taut and slippery.

Recipe: Decoction of Pinellia, White Atractylodes and Gastrodia

Rhizoma Pinelliae Praeparata	9 g
Rhizoma Atractylodis Macrocephalae	9 g
Rhizoma Gastrodiae	9 g
Pericarpium Citri Reticulatae	9 g
Poria cum Ligno Hospite	15 g
Radix Glycyrrhizae	6 g
Rhizoma Zingiberis Recens	6 g
Fructus Ziziphi Jujubae	7 pcs

All the above drugs are to be decocted in water for oral administration.

3. Deficiency of both Spleen and Kidney

Main Symptoms and Signs: There are repeated occurences of vertigo and tinnitus which is like singing of cicadas, accompanied with short breath, fatigue, soreness and weakness of the waist and knees, amnesia, excessive dreaming during sleep, clear urine and long-time urination at night, reddish tongue with white fur, and thready and feeble pulse.

Therapeutic Principle: Replenishing qi, warming the kidney and removing water retention to relieve dizziness.

Recipe: Decoction for Reinforcing Middle-jiao and Replenishing qi, compounded with Diuretic Decoction by Strengthening Yang of the Spleen and Kidney

Radix Astragali seu Hedysari	24 g
Radix Ginseng	9 g
Rhizoma Atractylodis Macrocephalae	9 g
Pericarpium Citri Reticulatae	9 g
Rhizoma Cimicifugae	9 g
Radix Bupleuri	9 g
Radix Aconiti Praeparata	9 g

Rhizoma Zingiberis Recens	9 g
Radix Angelicae Sinensis	15 g
Poria cum Ligno Hospite	15 g
Radix Paeoniae Alba	15 g
Radix Glycyrrhizae	6 g

All the above drugs are to be decocted in water for oral administration.

For those who have excessive liver-fire, add 9 grams of Radix Gentianae and 9 grams of Cortex Moutan Radicis. For those who have severe tinnitus, add 9 grams of Magnetitum and 9 grams of Rhizoma Acori Graminei. For those suffering from insomnia and dysphoria, add 15 grams of Caulis Polygoni Multiflori, 15 grams of Os Draconis Fossilia Ossis Mastodi and 15 grams of Concha Ostreae. For those with severe nausea and vomiting, add 15 grams of Haematitum, 9 grams of Flos Inulae (wrapped in a piece of gauze before it is decocted) and 6 grams of Caulis Bambusae in Taeniam.

4. Deficiency of Qi and Blood

Main Symptoms and Signs: Vertigo accompanied by pallor and lustreless complexion, short breath, palpitation, insomnia, pale lips and nails, lassitude, pale tongue, thready and weak pulse.

Therapeutic Principle: Replenish qi and blood.

Recipe:

Radix Codonopsis Pilosulae	15 g
Radix Astragali seu Hedysari	30 g
Rhizoma Atractylodis Macrocephalae	12 g
Pericarpium Citri Reticulatae	9 g
Rhizoma Cimicifugae	9 g
Radix Bupleuri	9 g
Radix Angelicae Sinensis	12 g
Radix Paeoniae Alba	15 g
Radix Glycyrrhizae Praeparata	6 g

All the above drugs are to be decocted in water for oral administration.

Patent Medicine: Angelica blood-supplementing pill (Danggui yangxue wan). Take 9 g, twice daily.

Chapter Twenty-one
Hysteria

Hysteria is a common type of neuroses, occurring more often in young women. The disease is characterized by delusion of grnadeur, mannerism, sensitive to hint etc.. Attacks of this disease is often due to mental factors. It belongs to the categories of "Zang Zao", "lily disease" and "melancholia" in traditional Chinese medicine.

I. DIFFERENTIATION

1. Liver-qi Depression: Distress of the chest and sighing, fullness or distending pain in the hypochondria, aggravated by anger, thin and white tongue coating, deep and taut pulse.

2. Insufficiency of Blood: Trance, grief and anger without reasons, irritability, difficulty in self-control, palpitation, listlessness, pale tongue with thin and white coating, taut and thin pulse.

II. TREATMENT

1. Body Acupuncture

Prescription: Shuigou(DU26), Hegu(LI4), Taichong(LR3).

Supplementary points: For liver-qi stagnation, Yanglingquan(GB34) and

Shanzhong(RN17) are added; for insufficiency of blood, Jiuwei(RN15) and Neiguan(PC6).

Method: Use filiform needles to puncture the points with reducing method.

2. Auricular Acupuncture

Prescription: Gan(CO12) liver, Xin(CO15) heart, Shenmen(TF4) shenmen, Pizhixia(AT4) subcortex, Jiaogan(AH6a) sympathetic nerve, Zhen(AT3) occiput.

Method: Use filiform needles to puncture the points with strong twirling and rotating method for continuous five minutes and retain them for 30 to 40 minutes. The needles are not withdrawn until the symptoms disappear and the patient feels easy.

Chapter Twenty-two
Hyperkinetic Syndrome of Childhood（MBD）

Hyperkinetic syndrome of childhood, also called minimal brain dysfunction syndrome, is an illness commonly seen in school-age children. It is clinically characterized by a divided attention, hyperactivity, incoordination, difficulty in learning but normal mental ability in most cases. The incidence is 5% to 10%, more often found in boys than in girls. It affects the children's study and life, school education and family spirit. Recently paediatricians, neuropathists, psychiatrists and psychologist at home and abroad have paid great attention to the treatment and education of the sick children.

I. ETIOLOGY AND PATHOGENESIS

1. Congenital Factor. A fetus originates from the reproductive essence of the parents. In case of deficiency of the essence, the fetus will not be well nourished; in case of consanguineous marriage, yin and yang of the fetus will be both deficient. Furen Liangfang Daquan points out, "balanced yin and yang make the body perfect". Unbalanced yin and yang make zang and fu fail to be well nourished, causing dysfunction of , especially, the heart, spleen, liver and kidney. The growth and development of the fetus are affected, resulting in hyperkinetic syndrome.

The balance of yin and yang is essential for keeping health and mental acitivities. Yinyang Yingxiang Dalun says, "Yin exhibits serenity and tranquility while yang exhibits impetuousness and restlessness." and "Yin exhibiting the inside is the material basis of yang while yang exhibiting the outside is the manifestation of the function of yin. They are relate to each other". Alternate activity and inertia are based on the balance of yin and yang. The hyperkinetic children mainly present with deficiency syndrome, characterized by yin-deficiency due to excess of yang activity and yang floating in the exterior due to failure of yin to control yang.

The dysfunction of zang and fu organs mainly means the dysfunction of the heart, spleen, liver and kidney. The heart governs blood circulation and spirit. The sound of the heart is speech. Pu Ji Fang says, "Heart, the home of spirit, the source of intelligence, should always stay quiet." It means that all mental activities originate from the heart. The mind will work well after the heart is well nourished. Heart belongs to fire, or yang. The excessive activities of the heart would cause disease. In childhood, yang is usually excessive and heart-fire is apt to be hyperactive. If heart-yin is deficient, the heart will not be well nourished by blood supply, the spirit is out of order, and the mental ability will be poorly developed. It is manifested by hyperactivity, a short attention span, language difficulty and inability to learn. Spleen is an organ in charge of yin. Dysfunction of the spleen is often seen in childhood. Poor nursing, improper diet, indigestion will cause insufficiency of the spleen and that will result in thinking and emotional problems, changeable interests, speaking without due consideration. The liver, one of the Zang organs, is firm and active in character. It is in charge of the tendons and soul- storing. It is related with rage and temperament. In children liver-qi is often overabundant. In case of deficiency of liver- yin and hyperactivity of liver-yang, irritability, impulsivity and stubbornness, shouting and hyperactivity may be found in the suffers. Being the origin of congenital constitution, kidney stores vital essence with the ears as its window, which nourishes the brain and the marrow. If kidney can not dominate the vones and forms marrow because of deficiency of kidney- yin, the brain and marrow will be insufficient, showing clumsy and awkward, incoordination, poor power of recognition and listening, and enuresis. Besides, liver-yang is liable to be hyperactive because of deficiency of the kidney-yin and heart fire is excessive because kidney water is not able to control fire. Deficiency of spleen-qi will give rise to accumulation of dampness and phlegm which attack the heart and mind, resulting in mental retardation.

2. Acquired Factor. Difficult delivery, anoxia, asphyxia, head injury (hemorrhge, traumata), cerebral diseases (cerebritis, meningitis) can all cause the injury of channels, leading to outflow or stagnation of blood and qi, obstruction of orifices or channels, disturbance of the spirit. Thus appear reslessness, activeness and irritability.

In addition, the development of the disease has something realted to the family, environment, education and diet.

II. MAIN POINTS OF DIAGNOSIS

1. Historical Data. Perhaps it is related to heradity, difficult delivery, anoxia, asphyxia, head injury (hemorrhage, traumata), infection (cerebritis, meningitis), family environment and education, etc..

2. Main Symptoms and Signs

1) Dyskinesia. Overactive behavior is evident and purposeless and shifts from moment to moment. The sick child fails to keep prolonged attention on a given task, characterized by distraction, hand-shaking, tongue-extending, eye-making, difficulty to sit quiet, clumsy and incoordination.

2) Behavior Disorder. Inpulsivity, uncontrollable rage, temper and tantrum may be seen in the patient. He may be against the rules, tell lies, fight with others frequently, fail to control himself.

3) Learning Problems. The child show distraction with unsteady studying marks.

3. Neurologic Examination. There are not any evident postive signs. The mental ability may be normal. There is minimal brain dysfunction such as clumsyness, mild ataxia, slow finger-to- finger test and turning hand-test.

4. Electroencephalography (EEG). EEG is without any specificity. It may be normal. There will be a slight diffuse dysrythmia.

III. DIFFERENTIATION AND
TREATMENT OF COMMON SYNDROMES

In addition to giving medicine therapy, the doctor, cooperated by the teachers and parents, should patiently educate and direct the sick child for his abnormal psychologic and behavior problems. First correct abnormal behavior that is not very serious, encourage him to have confidence and to set up new behavior gradually.

1. Deficiency of Yin Leads to Hyperactivity of Yang due to Deficiency of Liver-Yin and Kidney-Yin

Main Symptoms and Signs: Emaciation, flushed face, dysphoria with feverish sensation in the chest, palms and soles, distraction, hyperlogia and hyperactivity, restlessness and irritability, sometimes enuresis; red and dry tongue with thin fur, d wiry, small and rapid pulse.

Therapeutic Principle: Nourishing yin and suppressing the excessive yang, relieving mental stress

Recipe: Zuogui Wan (Zuogui Bolus), modified.

Rhizoma Rehmanniae Praeparata	9 g
Rhizoma Diocoreae	9 g
Cortex Moutan Radicis	9 g
Plastrum Testudinis	9 g
Radix Paeoniae Alba	9 g
Os Draconis	15 g
Concha Ostreae	15 g
Radix Polygalae	9 g
Rhizoma Acori Graminei	12 g
Fructus Schisandrae	6 g
Fructus Alpinae Oxyphyllae	12 g
Fructus Lycii	12 g
Radix Glycyrrhizae	3 g'

All the above drugs are to be decocted in water for oral administration.

It can also be made into water-paste pill or honey-paste pill or mixture. It is to be taken for 2 to 3 month.

Modification: Additional Semen Cuscuta 12 g, Ootheca Mantidis 9 g, Fructus Rosae Laevigatae 9 g should be given in case of enuresis. In case of epilepsy-like fit, refer to infantile epilepsy.

2. Floating Yang Acts Recklessly due to Qi Deficiency of the Heart and Spleen.

Main Symptoms and Signs: Pale complexion, restlessness, changeable interests, divided attention, amnesia, dreaminess, stutter or problem in formation of phrases and sentences, redness on both sides and the tip of the tongue with whitish coating, thready and feeble pulse or thready and rapid pulse.

Therapeutic Principles: Nourishing the heart to calm the mind, restoring qi to add wisdom.

Recipe: Guipi Tang (Decoction for Invigorating Spleen and Nourishing Heart) and Gan Mai Dazao Tang (Decoction of Radix Glycyrrhizae, Fructus Tritici Levis and Fructus Ziziphi Jujubae), modified.

Radix Pseudostellariae	12 g
Poria	9 g
Rhizoma Atractylodis Macrocephalae	9 g
Radix Angelicae Sinensis	9 g
Radix Astragali seu Hedysari	12 g
Radix Polygalae	9 g
Semen Ziziphi Spinosae	9 g
Rhizoma Acori Graminei	9 g
Fructus Schisandrae	6 g
Fructus Ziziphi Jujubae	10 grains
Fructus Tritici Levis	15 g
Radix Glycyrrhizae	6 g

All the above drugs are to be decocted in water for oral administration.

Modification: Ramulus Uncariae cum Uncis 9 g, Dens Draconis 12 g, Concha Margaritifera Usta 15 g should be added in case of dreaminess or sleep-walking. Radix Polygalae 9 g, Os Draconis Fossilia 12 g, Rhizoma Acori Graminei 12 g should be added for those who have amnesia.

3. Retention of Damp Heat in the Interior; Disturbance of Interior by Phlegm and Heat.

Main Symptoms and Signs: Chest tightness, loss of appetite, thirst, red lip and foul breath, abundant expectoration and bitter taste, constipation and yellow urine, hyperlogia and hyperactivity, spiritual laxity, changeable emotion, greasy and yellowish fur, smooth and rapid pulse.

Therapeutic Principle: Cleaning away phlegm, quenching pathogenic fire and calming the mind.

Recipe: Huanglian Wendan Tang (Decoction of Rhizoma Coptidis to Warm the Gallbladder), modified.

Rhizoma Pinelliae Praeparata	9 g
Pericarpium Citri Reticulatae	9 g
Poria	12 g
Cortex Magnosiae Officinalis	9 g
Radix Curcumae	9 g
Rhizoma Acori Graminei	12 g
Talcum	9 g
Fructus Aurantii	9 g
Fructus Forsythiae	12 g
Rhizoma Coptidis	6 g
Radix Glycyrrhizae	3 g

All the above drugs are to be decocted in water for oral administration.

4. Unnourished Orifices due to Obstruction of Channels Caused by Blood Stasis

Main Symptoms and Signs: In addition to hyperkinetic symptoms, the children have a history of birth injury and intracranial hemorrhage, dark and gloomy complexion, rage for nothing, dark red tongue and uneven pulse.

Therapeutic Principles: Promoting blood circulation by removing blood stasis; relieving mental stress and inducing resuscitation.

Recipe: In addition to the above-mentioned ingredients, Radix Paeoniae Rubra 9 g, Radix Saliva Miltiorrhizae 12 g, Flos Carthami 6 g are added.

IV. OTHER THERAPIES

1. Acupuncture Therapy

Choose points according to the rules of relieving mental stress, calming the liver and supressing yang, strengthening the mind and calming the mind, regulating the flow of qi and relieving depression.

Main Points: Neiguan(PC6), Taihcong(LR3), Dazhui(DU14), Quchi

(LI11).

Adjunct Acupuncture Points: Baihui(DU20), Sishencong(EX-HN1), Daling(PC7) for the unconscious. Anshen(EX), Anmian(EX), Xinshu(BL15) for overactivity. Shenting(DU24), Shanzhong(RN17), Zhaohai(KI6) for reslessness.

Manipulation: Quick and deep inserting. After insertion, tap Jiaji(EX-B2), Urinary Bladder Meridian, Du Channel with plum- blossom needle to the extent of the skin until it becomes red. Once every two days. In older children, electric stimulator can be used.

2. Auricular Plaster Therapy

Points: Pizhixia (AT4) subcortex, Naogan (AT3, 4i) brain stem, Shen (CO10) kidney.

Method: Semen Vaccariae or Semen Ziziphi Spinosae are applied tightly to the particular points and renew them twice a week, press them half to one minute, three times daily. Two ears are in shifts. Fifteen shifts consisted of one course of treatment, with a 14-day interval between courses.

V. PREVENTION AND NURSING

1. Pay attention to perinatal care. Prevent difficult labor and baby's head injury.

2. Teahcers and parents should not blame, beat and is criminate against the sick children. Patiently help them, and make them encouraged to correct their wrong behaviors gradually. Their minor improvement should be praised and encouraged.

Chapter Twenty-three
Schizophrenia

Schizophrenia is the most common psychosis. Its etiology has not been well understood despite many years of studies. Generally, genetic and environmental factors are considered to be involved in causing the disease. Schizophrenia frequently occurs in young adults. The ratio of incidence between males and females is roughly equal. In traditional Chinese medicine, this disease is included in the categories of "Yu Zheng" (melancholia), "Dian" (depressive psychosis), "Kuang" (mania), etc..

I. MAIN POINTS OF DIAGNOSIS

1. Most patients have distortion, introversion, sensitiveness, doubting mania, fantasy and other features before the attack, which are associated with weak neural type.

2. The major psychogenic symptoms include obstacle of thinking (split of thought and incoherence of thinking), obstacles of affect and volition. Delusion is a common symptom and may become a noticing manifestation. Auditory and visual hallucination and depersonalization may appear in some patients.

3. Clinically, the disease can be divided into different types according to their manifestations: simple type, hebephrenic type, catatonic type and paranoid type. The last is the most common of all.

4. The general physical examination, nervous examination and tests of

blood, urine and stool show no abnormal changes. Diagnosis depends chiefly on the history of the illness and symptoms.

II. DIFFERENTIATION AND TREATMENT OF COMMON SYNDROMES

1. Syndrome of Depressive Psychosis (Stagnancy of Phlegm and Qi)

Main Symptoms and Signs: Emotional depression, apthy, dementia, divagation or mutter to oneself, frequent cry or laugh for no apparent reason, caprice, no desire for diet, white greasy coating of the tongue, taut and slippery pulse.

Therapeutic Principles: Resolving phlegm, alleviating mental depression and regulating the flow of qi to treat psychosis.

Recipe: Modified Decoction for Regulating the Flow of Qi and Expelling Phlegm.

Pericarpium Citri Reticulatae	10 g
Rhizoma Pinelliae	10 g
Poria	10 g
Radix Glycyrrhizae	6 g
Arisaema cum Bile	10 g
Fructus Aurantii Immaturus	10 g
Radix Polygalae	10 g
Rhizoma Acori Graminei	10 g
Rhizoma Cyperi	10 g
Radix Curcumae	12 g

All the above drugs are to be decocted in water for oral administration.

Besides, 10 grams of Radix Coptidis are to be added for the case with restlessness, yellowish coating of the tongue and rapid pulse; and 10 grams of Radix et Rhizoma Rhei added for constipation; 12 grams of Semen Ziziphi Spinosae, 10 grams of Dens Draconis and 30 g of Magnetitum for insomnia. If the patient's

· 144 ·

depressive psychosis lasts for a long time resulting in loss of qi and blood of the heart and spleen, with the symptoms of palpitation, insomnia dreaminess and trance, 10 grams of Radix Codonopsis Pilosulae, 10 grams of Radix Angelicae Sinensis, 10 grams of Radix Salviae Miltiorrhizae and 10 grams of Semen Ziziphi Spinosae supplemented.

2. Syndrome of Manic Psychosis (Flaring up of Phlegm-Fire)

Main Symptoms and Signs: Sudden onset, irritability, flushed face, blood-shot eyes, mania, restlessness, constant scolding and beating, climbing up to a high place and singing, unusual strength, anorexia and insomnia, red tongue with yellow and greasy fur, slippery and rapid pulse.

Therapeutic Principle: Purging liver-fire, tranquilizing the mind and removing phlegm.

Recipe: Modified Prescriptions of Pill for Removing Phlegm and Pig Iron Cinder Drink

Lapis Chloriti	20 g
Radix et Rhizoma Rhei	10 g
Radix Scutellariae	12 g
Radix Coptidis	10 g
Radix Gentianae	10 g
Fructus Aurantii Immaturus	10 g
Rhizoma Pinelliae	10 g
Arisaema cum Bile	10 g
Rhizoma Acori Graminei	10 g
Concretio Silicea Bambusae	10 g

All the above drugs are to be decocted in water for oral administration.

If the patient suffers from mania for a long period of time, excessive fire will hurt yin, which is manifested as restlessness and easy scare, emaciation, flushed face, red tongue, fine and rapid pulse. In such a case the above recipe should include dried Radix Rehamnniae 15 g, Radix Ophiopogonis 10 g and Radix Scrophulariae 12 g.

Patent Medicine: Pill for Removing Phlegm (chlorit phlegm- expelling pill). Take one pill, three times daily.

III. ACUPUNCTURE AND MOXIBUSTION THERAPY

1. Body Acupuncture

Main Point: Fenglong(ST40).

Complementary Points: Add Xinshu (BL15), Ganshu (BL18), Pishu (BL20) and Shenmen (HT7) for depressive disorder; Shuigou (DU26), Shaoshang(LU11), Yinbai(SP1), Fengfu(GB16), Daling(PC7) and Quchi (LI11) for manic disorder.

Method: Use filiform needles to puncture the points with the even manipulation for the depressive disorder, with reducing method for manic disorder.

2. Electrotherapy

Prescribed Points: Shuigou(DU26), Baihui(DU20), Dazhui(DU14), and Fengfu(GB16).

Method: 2 points are used for each treatment. The needles are connected with the pulse current after the insertion of the needles and arrival of qi for 5 to 20 minutes. A strong and long stimulation is used for the manic disorder, while a strong, intermittent and short stimulation for the depressive disorder.

Chapter Twenty-four
Recipes for Treating
Neurogenic and Psychogenic Diseases

Acanthopanax Infusion
(Wujiashen Chongji)

Ingredients:

Radix Acanthopanacis Senticosi

Process: Make medicinal cubes (infusion), 25 g each cube.

Actions: Strengthening the body resistance and restoring normal functions of the body to consolidate the constitution, relieving mental stress and promoting intelligence.

Indications: Insomnia, excessive dreaming, fatigue and weakness, poor appetite and others caused by neurosis and other diseases. It has certain effects in relieving angina pectoris of coronary heart disease. It is also used for the treatment of leukopenia.

Direction: To be taken orally after being infused in boiling water, one cube each time, twice daily.

Banlong Pill
(Ban Long Wan)

INGREDIENTS:

Colla Cornu Cervi	10 g
Poria	10 g
Semen Biotae	10 g

Semen Cuscutae	10 g
Fructus Psoraleae	10 g
Pulvis Cornu Cervi	20 g
Radix Rehmanniae Praeparata	20 g

EFFICACY: Nourishing and invigorating the kidney-essence, preserving sperm and tranquilizing; mainly for cases of nocturnal emission, impotence or premature ejaculation accompanied with lumbago, tinnitus, nocturia, dizziness, fatigue, pale complexion, pale tongue with white fur, sunken and small, weak pulse, which are attributive to the impairment of kidney-essence and weakness of kidney qi.

INDICATIONS: 1. Applicable to cases of prolonged metrorrhagia or leucorrhagia, accompanied with dizziness, lumbago, weakness of the knee joints, spiritlessness, pale tongue with whitish fur, feeble pulse, which are attributive to insufficiency of essential substance and blood and weakness of kidney qi. 2. For cases with spontaneous flow of thin breast milk after delivery, shortness of breath, fatigue, lumbago, dimmish complexion, pale tongue with whitish fur, sunken and feeble pulse, which are attributive to insufficiency of kidney-essence and deficiency of kidney qi. 3. Also applicable to cases of hypothyroidism, neurasthenia, Addison's disease, dysfunctional uterine bleeding, hysteromyoma and endometritis, which are attributive to insufficiency of essential substance and blood, and deficiency of kidney qi.

INTERPRETATION: Colla Cornu Cervi not only invigorates essential substance and blood but also warms and strengthens kidney yang, and serves as the principal drug of the prescription. Radix Rehmanniae Praeparata and Semen Cuscutae can benefit yin and invigorate yang, which tonifies the essential substances, blood and kidney-yang when it is used together with Colla Cornu Cervi. Fructus Psoraleae acts with Colla Cornu Cervi to invigorate kidney and strengthen yang. Semen Biotae used together with Poria serves to keep heart-fire and kidney-water in balance, and tranquilize the patient. Fructus Psoraleae enhances the emission-relieving effect of Cornu Cervi.

Baolong Pill
(Baolong Wan)

INGREDIENTS:

Concretio Silicae Bambusae	30 g
Realgar	3 g
Cinnabaris	15 g
Moschus	15 g
Rhizoma Arisaema cum Bile	120 g

PROCESS: Grind the above ingredients into powder to make pills.

EFFICACY: Clearing away heat, dispersing phlegm, relieving convulsion and fainting; mainly for infants with convulsive seizures attributive to accumulation of phlegm-heat, which manifest as fever, somnolence or loss of consciousness, rough breathing, convulsion, red tongue with yellow, turbid and greasy fur.

INDICATIONS: 1. Because the prescription contains Realgar and Moschus, it should not be boiled and prepared as decoction. 2. Applicable to infants with convulsion resulting from high fever, accompanied with red tongue and yellow fur, wiry and smooth pulse. 3. Also indicated for cases with epileptic seizures accompanied with yellow, turbid and greasy fur on the tongue, which are attributive to blockage of the orifices by phlegm-heat. 4. Also applicable to cases of uremic coma, hepatic coma and hysteria attributive to accumulation of phlegm-heat; and to cases of encephalitis B, epidemic meningitis, thermoplegia and cerebral malaria marked by high fever and convulsion, which are attributive to attack of severe heat and wind.

INTERPRETATION: Concretio Silicae Bambusae has the effects of clearing away heat, eliminating phlegm, cooling heart-fire and relieving convulsion. Arisaema cum Bile can disperse phlegm, suppress wind and relieve convulsion. The combination of two serves as the principal drugs for the treatment of convulsion of phlegm-heat type. Realgar can eliminate phlegm and toxic material. Moschus is used for waking up the patient from unconsciousness, and Cinnabaris for tranquilizing. The last three drugs together exert a strong anti-convulsive and resuscitating effect.

Bolus for Activating Meridians
(Huo Luo Dan)

INGREDIENTS:

Radix Aconiti Praeparata	6 g
Radix Aconiti Kusnezoffii Praeparata	6 g
Lumbricus	10 g
Rhizoma Arisaema cum Bile Praeparata	10 g
Olibanum	3 g
Myrrha	3 g

EFFICACY: Warming the channels, activating the circulation of collaterals, expelling wind evil, eliminating dampness and phlegm and removing blood stasis; mainly for cases with prolonged numbness and pain of the extremities, atttributive to retention of wind-phlegm and blood stasis in the meridians.

INDICATIONS: 1. Applicable to cases of arthralgia of wind- cold-dampness type manifested as prolonged immobility and pain of joints, numbness of muscles and skin, white and greasy fur on the tongue, wiry and smooth pulse. 2. Also applicable to cases of stroke attributive to obstruction of meridians by wind-phlegm, which are manifested as hemiplegia, spasm of limbs, white and greasy fur on the tongue and wiry pulse. 3. Also applicable to cases of Guillain-Barre syndromes, plexus brachialis neuralgia, ischialgia, multiple neuritis, etc., marked by pain of limbs, which are attributive to obstruction of meridians by wind-phlegm and blood stasis, or cases of reheumatic arthritis and cerebral accidents, which are attributive to attack of wind-cold-dampness or obstruction of the meridians by wind-phlegm.

INTERPRETATION: Radix Aconiti Praeparata and Radix Aconiti Kusnezoffii Praeparata can warm the channels, activate the circulation of collaterals and elimintae cold dampness evil from the meridians, and also expel wind evil and relieve pain. Rhizoma Arisaema cum Bile Praeparata can expel wind-phlegm from the meridians, relieve spasm and pain. The above three drugs constituent an effective remedy for eliminating wind-phlegm and blood stasis from meridians. Olibanum and Myrrha serve to disperse blood stasis from the meridians, and the wine can enhance their effects. Lumbricus is helpful to dredge and activate the meridians. In sum, the prescription aims at eliminating wind-phlegm and blood stasis from the meridians, and then relieving pain.

Bolus for Severe Endogenous Wind-Syndrome
(Da Ding Feng Zhu)

INGREDIENTS:

Radix Paeoniae Alba	18 g
Radix Rehmanniae	18 g
Colla Corii Asini	10 g
Radix Ophiopogonis	10 g
Plastrum Testudinis	12 g
Concha Ostreae	12 g
Carapax Trionycis	12 g
Semen Sesami	6 g
Fructus Schisandrae	6 g
Radix Glycyrrhizae Praeparata	3 g
Fresh egg yolk	1

EFFICACY: Nourishing yin and calming wind, mainly for cases of clonic convulsion attributive to damge of true-yin by heat and hyperactivity of liver-wind, which are accompanied with listlessness, crimson and uncoated tongue, small and weak pulse.

INDICATIONS: 1. Indicated for cases attributive to deficiency of liver-yin and kidney-yin and upward attack of liver-yang, which are manifested by dizziness aggravated by over strain or anger, soreness of the loin and knees, insomnia and dreaminess, nocturnal emission, fatigue, bright red tongue, small and rapid pulse. 2. Also applicable to cases of encephalitis B, epidemic meningitis, poliomyelitis and chorea, marked by convulsion, which are attributive to damage of true-yin by heat and hyperactivity of liver-wind.

INTERPRETATION: Egg yolk and Colla Corii Asini are applied to nourish yin-fluid, supplement the exhausted true-yin and calm liver-wind. Rehmanniae, Sesami, Ophiopogonis and Paeoniae Alba serve to nourish yin and blood, soothe the liver and calm wind. Plastrum Testudinis, Concha Ostreae and Carapax Trionycis can invigorate kidney-yin and suppress hyperactive liver-yang. Radix Glycyrrhizae Praeparata and Fructus Schisandrae are helpful for yin nourishing and wind calming.

Bolus of Arisaematis
(Tiannanxing Wan)

INGREDIENTS:

Arisaema cum Bile	10 g
Radix Angelicae Dahuriacae	10 g
Radix Ledebouriellae	10 g
Rhizoma et Radix Notopterygii	10 g
Radix Angelicae Pubescentis	10 g
Rhizoma Ligustici Chuanxiong	10 g
Rhizoma Gastrodiae	10 g
Radix Paeoniae Alba	10 g
Bombyx Batryticatus	10 g
Herba Ephedrae	6 g
Radix Platycodi	6 g
Herba Asari	6 g
Radix Glycyrrhizae Praeparata	6 g

Rhizoma Zingiberis	6 g
Borneolum Syntheticum	3 g
Moschus	0.6 g

PROCESS: All the above ingredients are to be prepared with honey as boluses.

EFFICACY: Expelling wind evil and phlegm, waking up the patient and dredging the meridians; mainly for cases of stroke attributed to accumulation of wind-phlegm evil in the interior, which are manifested as numbness of limbs, hemiplegia, aphasia, whitish and greasy fur on the tongue, floating and smooth pulse.

INDICATIONS: 1. Applicable to cases with swelling pain and immobility of joints, numbness of skin and muscle, whitish and greasy fur on the tongue, smooth pulse, which are attributed to artharalgia of wind-cold-dampness type. 2. Also applicable to cases of cerebral accidents, chronic rheumatic arthritis, sciatica, cervical vertebra syndrome, etc. manifested as hemiplegia, or arthralgia, or numbness of limbs, which are attributed to accumulation of wind-phlegm evil in the interior or arthralgia of wind-cold-dampness type.

INTERPRETATION: Arisaema cum Bile has a potent effect of expelling wind-phlegm evil and dredging the meridians, and acts as the chief drugs in the prescription. Bombyx Batryticatus enhances the effect of Arisaema cum Bile; Ledebouriellae, Notopterygii, Angelicae Pubescentis, Angelicae Dahuricae and Herba Menthae are helpful to expel wind evil and eliminate the dampness evil. Since phlegm-dampness evil is of yin nature, so Zingiberis and Asari are applied to warm the meridians and expel cold evil, and also help Arisaema cum Bile to dry the dampness and eliminate phlegm, so that the mobility of the extremities will be restored. Borneolum Syntheticum and Moschus have the effect of dredging the meridians, and are helpful to relieve aphasia. Gastrodiae, Glycyrrhizae Praeparata, Ligustici Chuanxiong and Paeoniae Alba have the effects of regulating vital energy and blood, subduing endogenous wind evil and relieving convulsion.

Bolus of Calculus Bovis for Purging Heart-Fire
(Niuhuang Qing Xin Wan)

INGREDIENTS:

Calculus Bovis	0.75 g
Cinnabaris	4.5 g
Rhizoma Copitidis	15 g
Radix Scutellariae	9 g
Fructus Gardeniae	9 g
Radix Curcumae	6 g

INDICATIONS: Clearing away heat evil and toxic material, waking up patients from unconsciousness by eliminating phlegm; mainly for seasonal febrile diseases with heat evil involving the pericardium and the phlegm-heat evil stagnating in the heart, which are manifested by high fever, irritability, coma, deliriu, red tongue with yellowish fur. Its action and indications are similar to but milder than "Bolus of Calculus Bovis Resurrection", and is suitable for the mild cases.

Bolus of Placenta Hominis
(Heche Ba Wei Wan)

INGREDIENTS:

Placenta Hominis	1 set
(cooked with ginger juice and wine),	
Fructus Corni	30 g
Radix Ophiopogonis	30 g
Radix Rehmanniae Praeparata	90 g
(cooked with ginger juice and Fructus Amomi)	
Cortex Moutan Radicis	15 g
Rhizoma Alismatis	15 g
Cornu Cervi Pantotrichum	60 g

Fructus Schisandrae	60 g
Rhizoma Dioscoreae	165 g
Poria	45 g
Radix Aconiti Praeparata	22 g
Ramulus Cinnamomi	22 g

PROCESS: Grind the above ingredients into powder to make pills with honey.

EFFICACY: Invigorating kidney, benefiting essence and vital energy and nourishing blood; mainly for cases attributive to impairment of kidney-energy and insufficiency of lung and spleen qi after epileptic seizures, which manifest as spiritlessness, dizziness, palpitation, lumbago, fatigue of the lower limbs, aversion to cold, weakness, poor appetite, loose stools, pale and corpulent tongue with white and smooth fur, slow and weak pulse.

INDICATIONS: 1. Indicated for infantile maldevelopment manifested by tardiness of ability to walk, delayed growth of the teeth, weakness of the tendon and bone, pale tongue with white fur, sunken and weak pulse, which are attributive to insufficiency of kidney-yang. 2. Also for cases of sterility, impotence or nocturnal emission accompanied with dizziness, tinnitus, lumbago, cold limbs, pale and corpulent tongue with white and smooth fur, which are attributive to the impairment of kidney-yang and insufficiency of essence and blood. 3. Applicable to cases of leukorrhagia with profuse thin discharge, lumbago, fatigue, feeling of coldness over the lower abdomen, nocturia, spiritlessness, which are attributive to the weakness of kidney qi and loss of essence fluid. 4. Also applicable to cases of senile dementia and climacterium syndrome with spiritlessness, which are attributive to the impairment of kidney qi and insufficiency of lung and spleen qi; and to cases of endometritis and senile vaginitis with leukorrhagia, which are attributive to weakness of kidney qi and loss of essence substance.

INTERPRETATION: The prescription is formed by adding Placenta Hominis, Ophiopogonis, Cornu Cervi Pantotrichum and Schisandrae to Pill for Invigorating Kidney Qi which has the effects of invigorating kidney yin, nourishing liver blood, benefiting spleen yin and strengthening kidney yang. Ophiopogonis and Schisandrae used together with the Boluses serves to nourish the lung and kidney. Cornu Cervi Pantotrichum is used for promoting the production of essence and marrow and benefiting qi. Placenta Hominis has a strong effect of tonifying qi and blood, and is available for various kinds of conscumptive diseases.

Bolus of Precious Drugs
(Zhi Bao Dan)

INGREDIENTS:

Cornu Rhinocerotis	30 g
Carapax Eretmochelydis	30 g
Succinum	30 g
Cinnabaris	30 g
Realgar	30 g
Borneolum Syntheticum	0.3 g
Moschus	0.3 g
Calculus Bovis	15 g
Benzoinum	45 g
Gold sheet	50 pcs (half for coating)
Silver sheet	50 pcs

PROCESS: All the above drugs are ground into powder and prepared into boluses, each weighs 3 g.

EFFICACY: Eliminating dampness-phlegm, waking up patients from unconsciousness, clearing away heart-fire and detoxifying; mainly for cases of coma, profuse expectoration, heavy breath, fever, restlessness, red tongue with yellowish, greasy and dirty fur, smooth and rapid pulse, which are attributive to the attack of the interior by heat evil and stagnation of dampness-phlegm, also for the infantile convulsion due to stagnation of phlegm- heat.

INDICATIONS: 1. Applicable to cases of sudden fainting or apoplexy attributive to the attack of pericardium by phlegm-heat although there is no fever. 2. Applicable to cases of sunstroke attributive to stagnation of dampness-phlegm and retention of summer-heat. 3. It has been recorded in Prescription of People' s Welfare Pharmacy that the bolus is taken with ginger juice to enhance the effect of waking up a patient. 4. Also applicable to comatose cases of hepatic coma, cerebrovascular accident, epilepsy, uremia, etc. which are attributive to retention of heat and dampness-phlegm.

INTERPRETATION: Calculus Bovis can eliminate phlegm, wake up one from unconciousness, clear away heart-fire and has the effect of detoxication. Its action is strong and rapid, so it is used as the principal drug. Moschu, Borneolum Syntheticum and Benzoinum have the effects of exorcising evils, dissipating dampness-phlegm and restoring consciousness; Cornu Rhinocerotis and Carapax Eretmochelydis can clear away heart-fire and have the action of detoxication. Realgar has the effect of detoxication and Cinnabaris, Succinum, gold sheet and silver sheet have the effect of tranquilizing. The combination of these drugs constitutes a prescription with eliminating dampness-phlegm and waking up one from unconsciousness as the chief effect, and with clearing away heart-fire and detoxifying as the auxiliary one. This is different from Bolus of Calculus Bovis for Resurrection.

Bolus of Storax
(Suhexiang Wan)

INGREDIENTS:

Rhizoma Atractylodis Macrocephalae	60 g
Radix Aucklandiae	60 g
Cornu Rhinocerotis	60 g
Rhizoma Cyperi	60 g
Cinnabaris	60 g
Fructus Chebulae	60 g
Lignum Santali	60 g
Benzoinum	60 g
Lignum Aquilariae Resinatum	60 g

Moschus	60 g
Flos Caryophylli	60 g
Fructus Pipers Longi	60 g
Borneolum Syntheticum	30 g
Oleum Storax	30 g
Olibanumm	30 g

PROCESS: All the above ingredients are prepared with honey to make boluses.

EFFICACY: Warming and dredging the meridians to wake up patients from unconsciousness, promoting the circulation of vital energy and eliminating the dampness evil; mainly for cases due to the obstruction of vital energy circulation by cold or phlegm- dampness evil and impairment of consciousness, which are manifested as sudden syncope, lockjaw, cyanosis and pallor, cold breath, whitish and smooth fur on the tongue, sunken, slow and strong pulse.

INDICATIONS: 1. Applicable to cases of angina pectoris attributive to stagnation of cold evil and vital energy or attack of dampness evil. 2. May be used as an emergency treatment for cases due to phlegm obstruction of the heart, manifested by epileptic seizures, mental upset, staring eyes, paraphasia, whitish and greasy fur on the tongue, before other causative treatments are applied. 3. Indicated only for cold type asthenia- syndrome of coma. 4. Also applicable to comatose cases of cerebral accidents, uremia, hepatic coma, etc.; mental disorders occuring in psychosis, such as schizophrenia, symptomatic psychosis, etc.; chest pain occuring in angina pectoris and myocardial infarction; which are attributive to the obstruction of vital energy circulation by cold or phlegm-dampness evil.

INTERPRETATION: This prescription is a typical prescription for waking up patient from unconsciousness, which composed of many aromatic drugs such as Storax, Benzoinum, Moschus and Borneolum Syntheticum, Cornu Rhinocerotis has the effects of clearing away heart-fire and eliminating toxic material; Cinnabaris, that of tranquilizing. The above six drugs used together are effective for waking up the patient from unconsciousness and for tranquilizing. Santali, Caryophylli, Cyperi, Aquilariae Resinatum, Pipers Longi, Boswelliae Olibanum and Atractylodis Macrocephalae constitute another group of herbs for regulating the function of viscera and enhancing the dampness-dispersing and waking effect.

Chebulae of warm and astringing nature is added to prevent the damage of healthy energy by the aromatic drugs.

Brain-Invigorating and Kidney-Tonifying Pill
(Jian Nao Bu Shen Wan)

INGREDIENTS:

Semen Ziziphi Spinosae

Radix Polygalae

Os Draconis Fossilia Ossis Mastodi

Radix Cyathulae

Cortex Eucommiae

Cinnabaris

Radix Angelicae Sinensis

Rhizoma Dioscoreae

Radix Ginseng

Cornu Cervi Pantotrichum

EFFICACY: Invigorating the brain, replenishing qi, tonifying the kidney and strengthening the essence of life.

INDICATIONS: Applicable to cases of neurosis, amnesia, insomnia, dizziness, vertigo, tinnitus, palpitation, lassitude in loin and knees, emission due to kidney deficiency, etc..

Cardiotonic Pill
(Tianwang Buxin Dan)

INGREDIENTS:

Radix Rehmanniae	120 g
Radix Scrophulariae	60 g
Radix Salviae Miltiorrhizae	60 g
Radix Angelicae Sinensis	60 g
Radix Ginseng	60 g
Poria	60 g
Semen Biotae	60 g
Semen Ziziphi Spinosae	60 g
Radix Polygalae	60 g
Radix Asparagi	60 g
Radix Ophiopogonis	60 g
Fructus Schisandrae	60 g
Radix Platycodi	60 g

DIRECTIONS: Take 9 grams three times daily. It can also be made into decoction, with the dosage modified proportionally according to the original recipe.

EFFICACY: Nourishing yin to remove heat and tonifying blood to tranquilize the mind.

INDICATIONS: 1. Asthenic fire stirring up inside due to deficiency of yin and blood brought on by the hypofunction of heart and kidney marked by insomnia with vexation, palpitation, mental weariness, nocturnal emission, amnesia, dry stools, orolingual boil, reddened tongue with little fur, thready and rapid pulse. 2. Neurosism, paroxysmal tachycardia, hypertension, hyperthyroidism and others marked by the above-mentioned symptoms can be treated by the modified recipe. 3. Modern researches have proved that the recipe has a better effect of regulating the cerebral cortex. It can tranquilize the mind to induce sleep without causing listlessness and achieve the effects of enriching the blood and relieving the symptoms of coronary heart disease.

CAUTIONS: The recipe is composed of nourishing, greasy drugs which affect the stomach, so it is not fit to take for a long time.

Decoction for Activating Blood Circulation
(Tong Qiao Huo Xue Tang)

INGREDIENTS:

Radix Paeoniae Rubra	10 g
Rhizoma Ligustici Chuanxiong	10 g
Semen Persicae	10 g
Bulbus Allii Fistulosi	10 g
Rhizoma Zingiberis Recens	10 g
Flos Carthami	6 g
Fructus Ziziphi Jujubae	6 pcs
Moschus	0.3 g
wine q. s.	

EFFICACY: Activating blood circulation and opening the orificies; mainly for cases of headache and dizziness due to accumulation of blood stasis in the head.

INDICATIONS: 1. Indicated for cases of alopecia, deafness and sinusitis, which are attributive to accumulation of blood stasis in the head. 2. For cases of sudden loss of vision which are attributive to accumulation of blood stasis in the eyes, omit wine and Ziziphi Jujubae and add Faeces Vespertilionis and Radix Salviae Miltiorrhizae to nourish blood and promote vision. 3. Also applicable to sequelae of cerebral concussion, cases of cerebral arteriosclerosis and cerebellar bleeding with headache and dizziness, and to cases of retinal hemorrhage and embolism of central retinal artery with sudden loss of vision which are attributive to the same mechanism.

INTERPRETATION: Persicae, Carthami, Paeoniae Rubra and Ligustici

Chuanxiong have the effects of activating blood circulation and removing blood stasis. Allii Fistulosi and Zingiberis help the above drugs distributing to the vertex. Moschus, fragrant and active, can dredge the passage of meridians and open the orifice, and is particularly suitable for the treatment of headache and dizziness due to accumulation of blood stasis in the head when used together with Persicae and Carthami. Wine and Ziziphi Jujubae used together have the effects of promoting blood flow and distributing the above drugs to the head.

Decoction for Clearing Heat in Ying System
(Qing ying Tang)

INGREDIENTS:

Cornu Rhinocerotis	2 g
Radix Rehmanniae	15 g
Radix Scrophulariae	9 g
Herba Lophatheri	3 g
Radix Ophiopogonis	9 g
Radix Salviae Miltiorrhizae	6 g
Rhizoma Coptidis	5 g
Flos Lonicerae	9 g
Fructus Forsythiae	6 g

All the above drugs are to be decocted in water for oral administration.

EFFICACY: Clearing and dispelling pathogenic heat from ying system, nourishing yin and promoting blood circulation.

INDICATIONS: Invasion of ying system by pathogenic heat manifested by feverish body which is aggravated in the night, delirium, insomnia due to vexation, or by faint skin rashes, deep-red and dry tongue and rapid pulse.

The recipe can also be modified to deal with ying-syndrome occuring in epidemic encephalitis B, epidemic cerebrospinal meningitis, septicemia and other infectious diseases.

INTERPRETATION: In the recipe, Cornu Rhinocerotis, being salty in flavour and cold in property, and Radix Rehmanniae being sweet in taste and cold in nature, both exert a role of a principal drug, having the effect of removing heat from ying and blood systems. Scrophulariae and Ophiopogonis together act as assistant drugs having the effect of nourishing yin and clearing heat. The rest share the role of adjuvant and guiding drugs. Lophatheri, Ophiopogonis, Lonicerae and Forsythiae are used to clear and dispel pathogenic heat from ying system through qi system, and Salviae Miltiorrhizae is used to promote blood circulation to remove blood stasis.

Clinically and Experimentally, it is ascertained that the recipe possesses the efficacies of relieving inflammation, bringing down fever, tranquilizing the mind, resisting bacteria and viruses, tonifying the heart, arresting bleeding, improving immunologic function, promoting blood circulation and so on.

Cases with white and slippery coating of the tongue which suggests invasion by pathogenic dampness should not use recipe in case it encourages pathogenic dampness.

Decoction for Eliminating
Dampness and Relieving Rheumatism
(Chu Shi Juan Bi Tang)

INGREDIENTS:

Rhizoma Atractylodis	12 g
Rhizoma Atractylodis Macrocephalae	10 g
Poria	10 g
Rhizoma seu Radix Notopterygii	10 g
Rhizoma Alismatis	10 g
Exocarpium Citri Grandis	6 g
Radix Glycyrrhizae	3 g
Succus Zingiberis	3 spoonfuls

Succus Bambusae   3 spoonfuls

EFFICACY: Strengthening the spleen, eliminating dampness, expelling wind, dissipating phlegm, relieving rheumatism and alleviating pain; mainly for cases of rheumatism manifested as localized arthralgia which will be aggravated in rainy days, fatigue, white and greasy fur on the tongue, wiry and smooth pulse, which are attributive to retention of dampness in the spleen and stomach and attack of wind-phlegm to the meridians and joints.

INDICATIONS: 1. For cases of apoplexy manifested by distortion of the face, dysphasia, numbness and spasms of limbs, or even hemiplegia, white and greasy fur on the tongue, wiry and smooth pulse, which are attributive to the attack of meridians by phlegm-dampness, omit Glycyrrhizae and add Scorpio, Bombyx Batryticatus. 2. For cases attributive to the attack of upper orifices by phlegm-dampness, which manifest as vertigo accompanied with nausea, vomiting, tinnitus, deafness, white and greasy tongue fur and wiry pulse, add Rhizoma Pinelliae Praeparata, Rhizoma Gastrodiae and omit Glycyrrhizae. 3. Also applicable to cases with rheumatic arthritis, sciatica and beriberi attributive to accumulation of dmapness in the spleen and stomach; to cases of facial paralysis, poliomyelitis and thromboangiitis obliterans of cerebral vessels with hemiplesia attributive to attack of meridians by wind-phlegm; and to cases of hypertension and cerebral arteriosclerosis, with dizziness attributive to attack of the upper orifices by phlegm-dampness.

INTERPRETATION: Atractylodis acts as the chief drug in the prescription and is applied in large dosage, which has the effects of activating the spleen, drying dampness, eliminating wind and alleviating pain. Atractylodis Macrocephalae and Poria serve to strengthen the spleen and promote diuresis. Citri Grandis can regulate vital energy and acitivate the spleen, thus assists in eliminating dampness. Succus Zingiberis and Lophatheri are used to expel wind, dredge meridians and dissipate phlegm.

Decoction for Hemiplegia
(Xu Ming Tang)

INGREDIENTS:

Lignum Cinnamomi	9 g
Radix Paeoniae Alba	9 g
Rhizoma Zingiberis	6 g
Herba Ephedrae	6 g
Rhizoma Ligustici Chuanxiong	6 g
Radix Codonopsis Pilosulae	6 g
Semen Armeniacae Amarum	6 g
Radix Angelicae Sinensis	9 g
Gypsum Fibrosum	15 g
Radix Glycyrrhizae	3 g

EFFICACY: Warming meridians, nourishing blood and expelling wind.

INDICATIONS: It is indicated for cases of hemiplegia after apoplexy, accompanied with weakness and rigidity of limbs, pale tongue with whitish fur, wiry and small pulse. Nowadays, it is usually applied for sequela of stroke. The action of this prescription is similar as that of the former, but its effect of warming meridians and strengthening yang energy is milder and has an additional effect of nourishing blood and expelling wind. It is suitable for cases of stroke attributive to deficiency of vital energy and blood and attack of the meridians by wind.

Decoction for Invigorating
Spleen and Nourishing Heart
(Gui Pi Tang)

INGREDIENTS:

Radix Astragali seu Hedysari	15 g
Radix Codonopsis Pilosulae	15 g
Radix Angelicae Sinensis	12 g
Arillus Longan	12 g
Rhizoma Atractylodis Macrocephalae	10 g
Poria	10 g
Semen Ziziphi Spinosae	10 g
Radix Aucklandiae	5 g
Radix Glycyrrhizae Praeparata	5 g
Radix Polygalae	3 g
Rhizoma Zingiberis Recens	5 pcs
Fructus Ziziphi Jujubae	5 pcs

INDICATIONS: Benefiting vital energy, strengthening spleen, invigorating the heart and nourishing blood; mainly for cases due to hypofunction of heart and spleen and insufficiency of vital energy and blood, manifested as palpitation, amnesia, insomnia, fatigue poor appetite, sallow complexion, or preceded menstrual cycle with profuse pale or continuously dripping discharge, pale tongue with whitish fur, small and weak pulse. For cases of metrorrhagia attributive to failure of the spleen to control blood, subtract Aucklandiae and polygalae and add Fructus Corni to nourish liver and stop metrorrhagia. For case with hematochezia attributive to hypofunction of spleen with retention of cold evil, subtract Polygalae and add Zingiberis Praeparata to warm middle jiao and stopping bleeding. Also applicable to cases of pepticulcer, dysfunctional uterine bleeding, thrombocytopenia purpura, aplastic anemia etc. with hemorrhage attributive to hypofunction of heart and spleen.

INTERPRETATION:　Astragali seu Hedysari and Codonopsis Pilosulae benefit vital energy and invigorate the spleen and serve as the chief drugs. Angelicae Sinensis and Arillus Longan tonify the blood, nourish the heart. The above four drugs used together strengthen both the heart and the spleen, and dealt with the primary aspect of the disease. Poria, Polygalae, Ziziphi Spinosae have the effects of nourishing the heart and calming the mental state, and dealt with the secondary aspect of the disease. Aucklandiae adn Atractylodis Macrocephalae strengthen the spleen adn regulate vital energy. Glycyrrhizae, Zingiberis Recens and Ziziphi Jujubae reconcile the action of spleen and stomach and promote the production of vital energy and blood. In summary, this prescription aims at benefiting vital energy and tonifying blood, when one's vital energy is sufficient, the heart is well nourished, the symptoms subside.

Decoction for Invigorating Yang
(Bu Yang Huan Wu Tang)

INGREDIENTS:

Radix Astragali seu Hedysari	60 g
Radix Angelicae Sinensis	15 g
Radix Paeoniae Rubra	15 g
Lumbricus	10 g
Rhizoma Ligustici Chuanxiong	10 g
Semen Persicae	6 g
Flos Carthami	6 g

EFFICACY:　Tonifying vital energy, promoting blood circulation and dredging the meridian passage; mainly for stroke sequelae such as hemiplegia, facial deviation, aphasia, slobbering, lower limbs paralyses, incontinence of urine, etc. with white fur and slow pulse.

INDICATIONS:　1. For cases of unconsciousness attributed to sthenia-syndrome, the therapy for waking up from unconsciousness should be applied before the prescription is given. 2. The purpose of using crude sample of Astragali seu Hedysari is to remove blood stasis, therefore, a large dosage (beginning from 30-60 g) should be applied in order to let it distributing all over the whole body. 3. For cases with much phlegm, add Rhizoma Arisaemacum Bile and Concretio Silicae Bambusae to eliminate the wind-phlegm; while for cases of aphasia, add Rhizoma Acori Graminei and Radix Polygalae to wake up the patient and eliminate phlegm. 4. For cases of bi-syndrome due to deficiency of vital energy and blood stasis, add Ramulus Taxilli to nourish the blood and eliminate wind evil. 5. The prescription may also be applicable to hemiplegia, paraplegia, monoplegia resulting from cerebrovascular accidents and infantile paralysis, and rheumatic arthritis, rheumatoid arthritis, etc. attributed to deficiency of vital energy and blood stasis.

INTERPRETATION: Astragali seu Hedysari is the principal drug in this prescription, while has the effect of tonifying vital energy to promote blood circulation. The other ingredients have the effects of promoting blood circulation and dredging the meridiean passage. The prescription, as a whole, can tonify vital energy and also promote blood circulation, remove blood stasis but not hurt the healthy energy. When the vital energy is sufficient, the blood flow activated, the blood stasis is removed and the meridian passage is dredged, all the above-metioned disorders will be relieved.

Decoction for Mild Hemiplegia
(Xiao Xu MIng Tang)

INGREDIENTS:

Lignum Cinnamomi	9 g
Radix Aconiti Praeparata	9 g
Radix Paeoniae Alba	9 g
Radix Ledebouriellae	9 g

Rhizoma zingiberis Recens	9 g
Herba Ephedrae	6 g
Rhizoma Ligustici Chuanxiong	6 g
Radix Codonopsis Pilosulae	6 g
Semen Armeniacae Amarum	6 g
Radix Scutellariae	6 g
Radix Stephaniae Tetrandrae	6 g
Radix Glycyrrhizae	3 g

EFFICACY: Warming meridians, promoting the motion of yang- energy, supporting healthy energy and eliminating wind; mainly for cases of hemiplegia accompanied with distortion of the face, aphasia, spasm of limbs, headache, rigid neck, whitish fur on the tongue, tense pulse, which are attributive to deficiency of healthy energy and attack of wind-cold to meridians.

INDICATIONS: 1. Applicable to rheumatism of wind-cold- dampness type with insufficiency of yang-energy, which manifests as wandering arthralgia, numbness of muscles and skin, limited movement of joints, white and smooth fur on the tongue, wiry and tense pulse. 2. This prescription is only suitable for stroke due to attack of the meridians by exogenous wind but contraindicated for cases of hemiplegia with distortion of the face of loss of consciousness which are attributive to impairment of liver and kidney, and the attack of asthenic wind inside the body. 3. Also applicable to cases of cerebral thrombosis and periodic paralysis with hemiplegia attributive to attack of meridians by wind-cold and to cases of chronic gouty arthritis, rheumatoid spondylitis, hyperplastic arthritis, etc. with arthralgia attributive to insufficiency of yang-energy and the attack of exogenous wind- cold-dampness.

INTERPRETATION: Ephedrae, ledebouriellae, Ligustici Chuanxiong and Armeniacae Amarum have the effects of dispelling superficial evils and warming and dredging meridians. Cinnamomi, Paeoniae Alba, Zingiberis Recens and Glycyrrhizae can regulate ying and wei, and not only enhance the effects of the above drugs but also increase the body resistance to defend against the attack of wind. Codonopsis Pilosulae and Aconiti Praeparata are used for benefiting vital energy and blood to restore the healthy energy and eliminate the evils when used with Paeoniae Alba and Ligustici Chuanxiong. Stephaniae Tetrandrae and Scutellariae can clear away the superficial heat and expel wind. Originally, there was Lignum Cinnamomi in the prescription, but it was often replaced by Ramulus Cinnamomi in the clinic. The former is good for warming the kidney to support yang, while the latter is for expelling wind, promoting sweating and warming and dredging the meridians. They may be applied accordingly.

Decoction for Removing
Blood Stasis in the Chest
(Xue Fu Zhu Yu Tang)

INGREDIENTS:

Radix Angelicae Sinensis	9 g
Rhizoma Ligustici Chuanxiong	5 g
Radix Paeoniae Rubra	9 g
Semen Persicae	12 g
Flos Carthami	9 g
Radix Bupleuri	3 g
Radix Platycodi	5 g
Fructus Aurantii	6 g
Radix Rehmanniae	9 g
Radix Glycyrrhizae	3 g
Radix Achyranthis Bidentatae	9 g

All the above drugs are to be decocted in water for oral administration.

EFFICACY: Promoting blood circulation to remove blood stasis and promoting circulation of qi to relieve pain.

INDICATIONS: 1. Syndrome of blood stasis in the chest marked by long-standing prickly chest pain and headache which exist in a certain region, or endless hiccup, dysphoria due to interior heat, palpitation, insomnia, irritability and liability to a fit of temper, running a fever gradually at dusk, deep-red tongue with ecchymoses, dark-purple lips or dark eyes, uneven pulse or taut and tense pulse. Coronary heart disease, cerebral thrombosis, thromboangiitis, obliterans, hypertension, cirrhosis of liver, dysmenorrhea, amenia, headache, chest pain and hypochondriac pain marked by stagnancy of qi and blood stasis can be treated by the modified recipe.

INTERPRETATION: The leading ingredients in the recipe are Radix Angelicae Sinensis, Rhizoma Ligustici Chuanxiong, Radix Paeoniae Rubra, Semen Persicae, Flos Carthami and Radix Bupleuri, which promote blood circulation to remove blood stasis. Among them, Radix Bupleuri also ensures proper downward flow of the blood. Radix Platycodi soothes the liver and regulates the circulation of qi. Fructus Aurantii and Radix Rehmanniae relieve the oppressed feeling in the chest, promote the circulation of qi to render blood circulation to be normal. Radix Achyranthis Bidentatae removes heat from the blood and combines Radix Angelicae Sinensis to enrich the blood and moisten dryness so as to remove blood stasis without impairment of yin. Radix Glycyrrhizae cooridinates the effects of all the other ingredients in the recipe.

Modern researches have proved that this recipe is especially effective in anticoagulation and antispasm. Besides, it has some effect on uterine contraction.

CAUTIONS: 1. Since this recipe is mainly composed of drugs for removing blood stasis, it should not be used to treat the syndrome without distinct stasis. 2. Contraindicated for pregnant cases.

Decoction for Sterility
(Hua Shui Zhong Zi Tang)

INGREDIENTS:

Radix Morindae Officinalis (soaked in salt solution)	10 g
Poria	10 g
Radix Codonopsis Pilosulae	10 g

Semen Cuscutae (fried with wine)	10 g
Semen Euryales (fried)	10 g
Rhizoma Atractylodis Macrocephalae (fried with earth)	12 g
Semen Plantaginis (fried with wine)	6 g
Cortex Cinnamomi	2 g

EFFICACY: Warming the kidney, strengthening the spleen and promoting diuresis, mainly for cases of sterility accompanied with lumbago, aversion to cold, cold limbs, fatigue, flat taste in the mouth, poor appetite, oliguria, edema of the lower limbs, puffiness of the body, corpulent tongue with white and greasy fur, sunken and slow pulse, which are attributive to deficiency of spleen-yang and kidney-yang, and retention of dampness in the uterus.

INDICATIONS: 1. Applicable to cases of impotence or nocturnal emission accompanied with dizziness, spiritlessness, lumbago, weakness of lower limbs, pale complexion, poor appetite, loose stools, pale tongue with white fur, sunken and slow pulse, which are attributive to declination of life-gate fire and deficiency of kidney-qi. 2. Also indicated for cases with general pitted edema which is more prominent in the lower part, lumbago, fatigue, cold limbs, aversion to cold, oliguria, poor appetite, loose stools, corpulent tongue with white smooth fur, sunken and slow pulse, which are attributive to deficiency of spleen-yang and kidney-yang and accumulation of cold-dampness in the interior. 3. Also applicable to cases of endocrine disorder such as hypothyroidism, and pelvic diseases such as endometritis with sterility attributive to deficiency of spleen-yang and retention of dampness in the uterus; to cases of hypogonadism and neurasthenia with impotence or nocturnal emission attributive to the declination of life-gate fire and deficiency of kidney-qi; and to cases of chronic nephritis with edema attributive to deficiency of spleen-yang and kidney-yang and accumulation of cold-dampness in the interior.

Decoction for Treating Rheumatism
(Juan Bi Tang)

INGREDIENTS:

Rhizoma seu Radix Notopterygii	10 g
Rhizoma Curcumae Longae	10 g
Radix Angelicae Sinensis (soaked with wine)	10 g
Radix Paeoniae Alba	10 g
Radix Ledebouriellae	10 g
Radix Astragalae seu hedysari	15 g
Radix Glycyrrhizae Praeparata	6 g
Rhizoma Zingiberis Recens	5 pcs

EFFICACY: Expelling wind and dampness, benefiting vital energy and nourishing blood; mainly for rheumatism of wind type attributive to the stagnation of wind-cold-dampness evil (predominantly the wind evil) in the meridians, which is manifested as immobility of the joints, wandering arthralgia, especially the neck, back, shoulder and elbow, thin and white fur on the tongue, floating and slow pulse.

INDICATIONS: 1. Applicable to cases of stroke manifested by deviation of the eyes and mouth, numbness of the muscles and skin, spasm of limbs, or hemiplegia (especially the upper limb), thin and whitish fur on the tongue, floating and wiry pulse, which are attributive to weakness of the superficies, deficiency of vital energy and attack of wind evil. 2. Also applicable to cases of rheumatic arthritis, rheumtoid arthritis, facial paralysis, cerebral accidents, etc., which are attributive to the stagnation of wind-cold-dampness evil (predominantly the wind evil) in the meridians.

INTERPRETATION: Nontopterygii and Ledebouriellae can expel wind evil, remove dampness evil and relieve pain, and is especially suitable for rheumatism of the upper body. Astragali seu Hedysari and Glycyrrhizae Praeparata have the effects of supplementing vital energy and strengthening the body surface and is helpful for expelling wind evil. Meanwhile, Astragali seu Hedysari and Glycyrrhizae Praeparata exert a tonifying effect without causing indigestion, and Notopterygii and Ledebouriellae promote vital energy circulation without losing it when all are used together. Angelicae Sinensis and Paeoniae Alba can nourish blood and promote blood circulation, Curcumae Longae is used for regulating vital energy in the blood; they are applied together for nourishing the blood to eliminate wind. Zingiberis Recens helps Notopterygii and Ledebouriellae to expel wind and dampness, and also helps Astragali seu Hedysari and Glycyrrhizae Praeparata to cooridinate ying-qi and wei-qi. Therefore, the prescription are also suitable for bi-syndrome due to wind-cold-dampness evil, characterized by deficiency of both ying-qi and wei-qi.

Decoction of Aneglicae Pubescentis and Taxilli
(Duhuo Jisheng Tang)

INGREDIENTS:

Radix Angelicae Pubescentis	10 g
Cortex Eucommiae	10 g
Radix Achyranthis Bidentatae	10 g
Radix Gentianae Macrophyllae	10 g
Poria	10 g
Radix Ledebouriellae	10 g
Radix Angelicae Sinensis	10 g
Radix Codonopsis Pilosulae	10 g
Radix Paeoniae Alba	10 g
Ramulus Taxilli	18 g
Radix Rehmanniae	18 g
Lignum Cinnamomi	1.5 g

Rhizoma Ligustici Chuanxiong	6 g
Herba Asari	3 g
Radix Glycyrrhizae	3 g

EFFICACY: Expelling wind-dampness evil, relieving arthralgia, benefiting the liver and kidney, invigorating vital energy and blood; mainly for prolonged arthralgia of wind-cold- dampness type with hypofunction of liver and kidney and insufficiency of vital energy and blood, which is manifested by cold pain over the loin and joints, limited mobility and flaccidity of joints, or numbness, aversion to cold and desire for warmth, pale tongue with whitish fur, small and weak pulse.

INDICATIONS: 1. Applicable to cases of stroke manifested by hemiplegia, numbness, spasm of limbs, pale tongue with whitish fur, small and weak pulse, which are attributive to deficiency of both the liver and the kidney, and attack of wind evil to the meridians. 2. Also applicable to cases of chronic rheumatic arthritis, rheumatic sciatica, lumbar strain, prolapse of lumbar intervertebral disc, etc., marked by cold pain over the loin and knees, which are attributive to prolonged bi-syndrome with deficiency of both the liver and the kidney and insufficiency of vital energy and blood.

INTERPRETATION: Angelicae Pubescentis, Ledebouriellae and Gentianae Macrophyllae have the effects of expelling wind and dampness, Asari expels wind-cold evil from the yin-channel and eliminates wind-dampness evil from the muscles and tendons; the above three drugs used together exert an analgesic effect for rheumatism of wind-cold-dampness type evil and relieving pain. Prolonged rheumatism (attack of wind-cold-dampness evil) may aggravate the deficiency of liver and kidney, so Ramulus Taxilli, Achyranthis Bidentatae and Eucommiae are applied to tonify the liver and kidney, strengthen the tendons and bones, Codonopsis Pilosulae, Poria, Glycyrrhizae to invigorate healthy energy, and Rehmanniae, Angelicae Sinensis and Paeoniae Alba to nourish blood and activate blood circulation. Moreover, Ligustici Chuanxiong and Lignum Cinnamomi are added to warm and dredge the vessels and expel wind evil. In sum, the prescription serves as both symptomatic and causative therapy for arthralgia by supplementing vital energy and blood, invigorating liver and kidney, and eliminating wind.

Decoction of Bupleuri Adding
Os Draconis and Concha Ostreae
(Chaihu Jia Longgu Muli Tang)

INGREDIENTS:

Radix Bupleuri	10 g
Radix Sutellariae	6 g
Rhizoma zingiberis Recens	6 g
Radix Codonopsis Pilosulae	6 g
Ramulus Cinnamomi	6 g
Radix et Rhizoma Rhei	6 g
Poria	6 g
Rhizoma Pinelliae	6 g
Minium	1 g
Fructus Ziziphi Jujubae	3 pcs
Os Draconis	15 g
Concha Ostreae	15 g

HZ⫟EFFICACY: Regulating shaoyang, dispersing phlegm, tranquilizing, supporting healthy energy and eliminating evil; mainly for cases attributive to invasion of heat to shaoyang (liver and gallbladder), which manifest feeling of oppression over the chest and hypochondrium, restlessness, delirium, frightening, insomnia, fatigue, red tongue with yellow fur, wiry and rapid pulse, i. e., the simultaneous occurence of asthenia- and sthenia-syndrome, cold and heat-syndrome, as well as superficies- and interior-syndrome.

INDICATIONS: 1. Minium is a poinsonous drug and s hould not be taken more than 10 g at one time and not for a long period. Now it is usually replaced by Ferrum scale. 2. Applicable to cases of epilepsy accom panied with dizziness, fatigue, pale complexion, red tongue with white and greasy fur, wiry and smooth pulse, which are attributive to adverse rising of wind-phlegm with simultaneous occurence of asthenia- and sthenia-syndrome. 3. Also indicated for cases of tinnitus and deafness accompanied with profuse expectoration, bitter taste in the mouth, feeling of oppression over the chest and hypochondrium, dizziness, fatigue, red tongue with yellow fur, wiry and rapid pulse, which are attributive to the adverse rising of phlegm-fire from the liver and gallbladder, with simultaneous occurence of asthenia- and sthenia-syndrome. 4. Also applicable to cases of hyperthyroidism, schizophrenia and neurasthenia marked by palpitation, which are attributive to the invasion of heat to shaoyang (liver and gallbladder); and to cases of Meniere's syndrome and sequelae of cerebral concussion marked by tinnitus and dizziness, which are attributive to adverse rising of phlegm- fire from the liver, gallbladder, with simultaneous occurrence of asthenia- and sthenia-syndrome.

INTERPRETATION: The prescription is composed on t he basis of the Decoction of Bupleuri for Regulating Shaoyang , by adding Ramulus Cinnamomi, Rhei, Poria, Minium, Os Draconis, Concha Ostreae and omitting Glycyrrhizae from it. Bupleuri serves to eliminate the pathogens from the interior when it is used together with Ramulus Cinnamomi and to clear away the heat located between the superificies and the interior when it is used together with Scutellariae. Rhei can directly clear away the interior heat. Pinelliae, Zingiberis Recens and Minium disperse phlegm and eliminate accumulated heat. Os Draconis and Concha Ostreae act as sedative. Codonopsis Pilosulae, Ziziphi Jujubae and Poria are applied for strengthening the spleen, benefiting vital energy and supporting healthy energy. In sum, the prescription aims at eliminating pathogens both from the superficies and interior by applying drugs both cold and warm in ntaure, tonifying and purging as well as descending and ascending in action.

Decoction of Bupleuri and Puerariae
for Expelling Evil from Muslces
(Chai Ge Jie Ji Tang)

INGREDIENTS:

Radix Bupleuri	10 g
Radix Puerariae	10 g
Gypsum Fibrosum	10 g
Radix Scutellariae	6 g
Radix Paeoniae Lactiflorae	6 g
Rhizoma seu Radix Notopterygii	6 g
Radix Angelicae Dahuriae	6 g
Radix Glycyrrhizae	3 g
Radix Platycodi	3 g
Rhizoma Zingiberis Recens	3 pcs
Fructus Ziziphi Jujubae	3 pcs

EFFICACY: Expelling the evil from the superficies, lowering fever and clearing away the interior heat evil; mainly for common cold of wind-cold type with formation of heat, which is manifested by chilliness becoming milder and fever higher, headache, soreness of limbs, eyes pain, thin and yellowish fur on the tongue, floating and bounding pulse, etc..

INDICATIONS: 1. For cases of warm-type malaria manifested by high fever, mild chilliness, general aching, red tongue with yellowish fur, wiry and rapid pulse, omit Radix Glycyrrhizae and Radix Platycodi and add Fructus Tsaoko eliminate dampness. 2. For cases of heat-type arthralgia manifested by joint aching, fever, chilliness, yellowish and greasy fur on the tongue, omit Radix Glycyrrhizae and Radix Platycodi, and add Cortex Phellodendri and Ramulus Cinnamomi to eliminate dampness-heat, dredge the meridians and relieve pain. 3. Applicable to cases of wind-fire toothache manifested by toothache referring to the head, chilliness, red tongue with whitish fur, wiry pulse. 4. Also applicable to cases of influenza, trigeminal neuralgia, rheumatic arthritis, etc. which are attributive to heat formation by stagnation of cold.

INTERPRETATION: Bupleuri and Puerariae have the effects of expelling the evil from the superficies and lowering fever. Notopterygii and Angelica Dahuricae have the effect of expelling wind evil from the body surface. Scutellariae and Gypsum Fibrosum have the effect of clearing away the interior heat evil. Paeoniae Lactiflorae is helpful to regulate ying and clear away heat evil. Platycodi helps Bupleuri to expel evil. Zingiberis Recens, Ziziphi Jujubae and Glycyrrhizae regulate the function of ying and wei and then the middle jiao. Although this prescription composes of the drugs of cold nature as well as those of warm nature, but, as a whole, its cold nature is greater than warm nature. However, it is still a prescription of acrid flavour and cool nature, which expels wind-heat.

Decoction of Cimicifugae
and Astragali seu Hedysari
(Shengma Huangqi Tang)

INGREDIENTS:

Radix Astragali seu Hedysari	30 g
Radix Angelicae Sinensis	12 g
Rhizoma Cimicifugae	6 g
Radix Bupleuri	6 g

EFFICACY: Benefiting vital energy, lifting yang and activating vital energy; mainly for cases of dysuria attributive to dysfunction of vital energy, which manifest difficult and dripping urination, tiredness, shortness of breath, pale tongue, slow and weak pulse.

INDICATIONS: 1. For cases attributing to deficiency and collapes of vital energy and downward flowing of essential substance, which manifest prolonged discharge of rice-water like urine, pale complexion, fatigue, pale tongue and feeble pulse, add Fructus Corni to keep the essential substance. 2. for protracted cases of nocturnal emission or enuresis accompanied with listlessness, pale complexion, pale tongue, sunken and feeble pulse, which are attributive to deficiency of vital energy, add Fructus Schisandrae and Ootheca Mantidis to calm the mental state and astringe the essential substance (or urine). 3. Also applicable to cases of chronic prostatitis, neurasthenia, senile dementia, etc. with difficult urination or enuresis, which are attributive to dysfunction of vital energy.

INTERPRETATION: This prescription is developed from the Decoction for Strengthening Middle Jiao and Benefiting Qi which is mainly for collapse of middle-jiao energy and hypofunction of spleen and stomach. In the prescription, Astragalic seu Hedysari is applied together with Cimicifugae for supplementing vital energy and raising yang to restore with Cimicifugae for supplementing vital energy and raising yang to restore the normal function of vital energy. Angelicae Sinensis and Bupleuri can disperse the stagnated liver-energy. In sum, the purpose of this prescription is to lift up collapse vital energy and restore the normal urination.

Decoction of Cinnamomi
(Guizhi Tang)

INGREDIENTS:

Ramulus Cinnamomi	10 g
Radix Paeoniae Alba	10 g
Radix Glycyrrhizae Preparata	6 g
Rhizoma Zingiberis Recens	5 pcs
Fructus Ziziphi Jujubae	5 pcs

EFFICACY: Expelling the yingfen and weifen; mainly for superficies-asthenia syndrome due to attack of exogenous wind- cold evil, which is manifested by fever, headache, sweating, aversion to wind, thin and whitish fur on the tongue, floating and slow pulse.

INDICATIONS: 1. The prescription is also capable of regulating ying and wei, so it is applicable to the cases with mild fever and chilliness, sweating, and slow pulse during postpartum or convalescence, and the cases of morning sickness attributing to imbalance of ying and wei. 2. According to the original record, hot porridge should be taken immediately after intake of the decoction in order to promote sweating and arrest retching. It is necessary to take hot porridge when diaphoretic effects is required, but not necessary when the ying-wei regulating action is required. 3. By adding Radix Puerariae, another prescription named Decoction of Ramulus Cinnamomi with Puerariae is formed. It has the effects of expelling wind evil from the superficies, activating stomach-qi to promote upward distribution of body fluid. It is indicated for the cases due to attack of the superficies by wind evil, with impairment of body fluid distribution and under nourishment of channels, which are manifested by stiffness and pain of the neck and back, sweating and aversion to wind. 4. By adding Cortex Magnoliae Officinalis and Semen Armeniacae Amarum, another prescription named Decoction of Ramulus Cinnamomi with Magnoliae Officinalis and Armeniacae Amarum is formed. It has the effects of expelling evils from the superficies, lowering the adverse rising energy and relieving asthma, it is indicated for asthmatics with new affection of wind-cold evil, which manifested by dyspneic cough with thin frothy sputum, sweating, aversion to wind, whitish and moist fur on the tongue, floating and slow pulse, etc.. 5. By adding Os Draconis and Concha Osteae, another prescription named Decoction of Ramulus Cinnamomi with Os Draconis and Concha Ostreae is formed. It has the effects of regulating yin and yang as well as tranquilizing, and is indicated for nocturnal emission, dizziness, easy dropping of hairs and coldness of genitalia, which are attributive to imbalance of yin and yang.

INTERPRETATION: Cinnamomi is of acrid flavour and warm nature, which has the effect of eliminating superficial wind evil. Paeoniae Alba is of sour flavour and cold nature, which strengthen ying and yin in the interior. These two drugs in combination serves to regulate the function of ying and wei, so as to expel the superficial evils from the body surface and regulate function of internal organs. Zingiberis Recens and Ziziphi Jujubae are used to enhance the above two drugs' effect of regulating the function of ying and wei. The application of Glycyrrhizae here is for strengthening yang by combining with Cinnamomi, for nourishing yin by combining with Paeoniae Alba, and for regulating stomach-qi by combining with Zingiberis Recens and Ziziphi Jujubae. The prescription not only can support yang and benefit yin, but also can induce perspiration with acrid flavour and astringe with sour flavour. So the evil will be eliminated along with sweating and perspiration will be stopped when the evil is cleared away.

Decoction of Cinnamomi Aconiti
(Guizhi Fuzi Tang)

INGREDIENTS:

Ramulus Cinnamomi	12 g
Radix Aconiti Praeparata	10 g
Rhizoma Zingiberis Recens	10 g
Fructus Ziziphi Jujubae	8 pcs
Radix Glycyrrhizae Praeparata	6 g

EFFICACY: Expelling wind and dampness, warming meridians and eliminating cold; mainly for cases attributive to the attack of wind-cold-dampness to the muscles and meridians, and circulatory impediment of vital energy and blood, which manifest general aching, immovability of trunk and limbs, no thirst nor vomiting, white and greasy fur, floating and unsmooth pulse.

INDICATIONS: 1. Applicable to cases with a yang-deficiency constitution and affection of wind-cold, which manifest chilliness, fever, aversion to wind, sweating, headache, cold limbs, tiredness of somnolence, white and greasy fur, sunken and slow pulse. 2. Also indicated for cases with chest pain referring to the back, feeling of oppression over the chest, tiredness, white and greasy fur on the tongue, wiry and slow pulse, which are attributive to accumulation of cold-dampness. 3. Also applicable to cases of rheumatic arthritis, sciatic periomarthritis, etc. with chillness and fever attributive to yang-deficiency and affection of exogenous wind-cold; and to cases of emphysema, coronary heart disease, rheumatic heart disease, etc. with chest pain attributive to accumulation of wind-phlegm.

INTERPRETATION: Aconiti has the effects of warming the meridians and eliminating cold-dmapness from the meridians. They two act as the principal drugs of the prescription. Zingiberis Recens and Ziziphi Jujubae serve to regulate ying and wei and can warm the meridians and promote the circulation of vital energy and blood when they are used together with Cinnamomi.

Decoction of Cinnamomi, Glycyrrhizae, etc.
(Guizhi Gancao Longgu Muli Tang)

INGREDIENTS:

Ramulus Cinnamomi	10 g
Radix Clycyrrhizae Praeparata	15 g
Os Draconis	30 g
Concha Ostreae	30 g

EFFICACY: Warming heart-yang energy and tranquilizing; mainly for cases attributive to impairment of heart-yang, which manifest palpitation, irritability, spontaneous sweating, pale tongue with white and greasy fur, floating and slow, or slow pulse with irregular intervals.

INDICATIONS: 1. For cases attributive to severe deficiency of heart-yang, which manifest sweating, cold limbs, feeble and large or slow and weak pulse, add Radix Aconiti Praeparata to recuperate the depleted yang. 2. Applicable to cases of nocturnal emission with dizziness, fatigue, spiritlessness, reddish tongue, small and slow pulse, which are attributive to ineqilibrium between yin and yang. 3. Also applicable to cases of rheumatic heart disease, sinus bradycardia and atrioventricular block with palpitation, which are attributive to deficiency of heart-yang; and to cases of neurasthenia and hypogonadism with nocturnal emission, which are attributed to inequilibrium of yin and yang.

INTERPRETATION: Glycyrrhizae is used in a large dose in this prescription and serves particulary to relieve palpitation and irritability. In sum, this prescription aims chiefly at warming and promoting heart-yang. Palpitation and other symptoms mentioned above may subside when the heart-yang is restored.

Decoction of Cinnamomi,
Paeoniae and Aemarrhenae
(Guizhi Shaoyao Zhimu Tang)

INGREDIENTS:

Ramulus Cinnamomi	10 g
Radix Paeoniae Alba	10 g
Rhizoma Zingiberis Recens	10 g
Rhizoma Atractylodis Macrocephalae	10 g
Radix Anemarrhenae	10 g
Radix Ledebouriellae	10 g
Radix Aconiti Praeparata	6 g
Herba Ephedrae	5 g
Radix Glycyrrhizae	3 g

EFFICACY: Expelling wind and dampness, activating yang-energy, relieving arthralgia, regulating yin and clearing away heat, mainly for cases with severe and imgratory arthralgia with swelling and increased temperature of the affected joints, dizzines, fatigue, nausea, vomiting, emaciation, thin and yellow greasy fur on the tongue, rapid pulse, which are attributive to accumulation of wind and dampness with production of heat evil.

INDICATIONS: 1. This prescription is suitable for arthralgia of wind-dampness type with formation of heat. It is not indicated for those cases with severe heat which manifest high fever, thirst, red tongue with yellow and dry fur, smooth and rapid bounding pulse. 2. Applicable to cases of apoplexy involving the meridians manifested by hemiplegia, rigidity of limbs, dizziness, thin and yellow greasy fur on the tongue, wiry pulse, which are attributive to prolonged retention of wind and phlegm-dampness in the meridians with transformation of heat. 3. Also applicable to cases of chronic gouty arthritis, rheumatic arthritis, periomarthritis, etc. attributive to accumulation of wind- dampness with trnasformation of heat; and to cases of sequela of cerebrovascular accident and rheumatic cerebrovasculitis with hemiplegia, which are attributive to retention of wind and phlegm-dampness in the meridians.

INTERPRETATION: Ramulus Cinnamomi, Ledebouriellae, Ephedrae and Atractylodis Macrocephalae are used together to eliminate wind-dampness from both superficies and interior. Paeoniae Alba and Anemarrhenae have the effects of regulating yin and clearing away heat. Aconiti serves to activate yang-energy, expel dampness and alleviate pain when it is used together with Ramulus Cinnamomi, Paeoniae Alba and Anemarrhenae. It is noteworthy that drugs of both hot and cold or yin and yang nature are used simultaneously in the prescription, and their actions are promoted each other instead of antagonized.

Decoction of Coptidis
(Huanglian Tang)

INGREDIENTS:

Rhizoma Coptidis	10 g
Ramulus Cinnmomi	10 g
Rhizoma Zingiberis	10 g
Rhizoma Pinelliae	10 g
Radix Codonopsis Pilosulae	6 g
Radix Glyccyrrhizae Praeparata	3 g
Fructus Ziziphi Jujubae	6 pcs.

EFFICACY: Regulating cold and heat, regulating function of stomach and lowering down the adverse rising qi; mainly for cases attributive to heat in the chest and cold in the gastrointestine, which are manifested by feeling of heat and oppression over the chest, vomiting, abdominal pain, white and smooth fur on the tongue and wiry pulse.

INDICATIONS: 1. Applicable to cases of watery diarrhea with increased gurgling sounds, abdominal pain, nausea, vomiting, vexation, thirst, yellow and greasy fur, soft and floating, smooth pulse, which are attributive to dampness-heat of intestine and stomach. 2. Indicated for cases with a feeling of gas rushing up through the thorax to the throat from the lower abdomen, accompanied with irritability, dry mouth but without desire to drink, white and greasy fur on the tongue, wiry pulse, which are attributive to incoordination between the liver and spleen, cold and heat, ascending and descending action. 3. Applicable to cases of duodenal ulcer, acute gastroenteritis, cholecystitis, or diarrhea attributive to heat in the upper and cold in the lower, or stagnation of dampness-heat in the intestines and stomach; or cases of hysteria and gastroenteric neurosis marked by feeling of gas rushing upward to the chest, and thorax, which are attributive to incoordination between the liver and spleen.

INTERPRETATION: Coptidis serves to clear away heat from the chest, and Zingiberis to expel cold from the gastrointestine. their actions match with each other. Pinelliae can ease the middle jiao when used together with Coptidis, and can regulate stomach and spleen and stop vomiting when used together with Zingiberis. Ramulus Cinnamomi serves to warm the middle jiao and expel cold when used together with Zingiberis and to regulate vital energy and lower down the adverse rising qi when used together with Pielliae. Codonopsis Pilosulae, Glycyrrhizae Praeparata and Ziziphi Jujubae calm the middle jiao and regulate the function of spleen and stomach. In sum, the prescription aims at regulating cold and heat, especially at warming middle jiao and expelling cold.

Decoction of Coptidis and Colla Corii Asini
(Huanglian E'jiao Tang)

INGREDIENTS:

Rhizoma Coptidis	10 g
Radix Scutellariae	10 g
Colla Corii Asini	12 g
Radix Paeoniae Alba	12 g
Fresh egg yolk	

EFFICACY: Clearing away heart-fire and nourishing kidney-yin; mainly for cases attributive to damage of true-yin by the heat evil entering shaoyin and hyperactivity of heart-fire, which are manifested by vexation, sleeplessness, feverish sensation over the body, palms and soles, dry mouth and throat, oliguria with yellow urine, red or crimson tongue with yellow fur, small and rapid pulse.

INDICATIONS: 1. For cases with fresh blood in the stool, irritability, dry throat, bitter mouth, red tongue with yellow fur, small and rapid pulse, which are attributive to excess of yang-qi and deficiency of yin-qi, and damage of the vessels by heat, use Radix Rehmanniae instead of egg yolk to cool the blood, sop bleeding and nourish yin-fluid. 2. Also applicable to cases of hyperthyroidism, diabetes mellitus, hypertension, neurasthenia, etc. with insomnia or nocturnal emission, and cases of nonspecific proctitis, tuberculous ulceration of rectum, chronic bacillary dysentery, etc., with bloody stool, which are attributive to excess of yang-qi and deficiency of yin-qi. 3. For cases with nocturnal emission or praecox ejaculation accompanied with dizziness, irritability, insomnia, oliguria with yellow urine, re tongue, small and rapid pulse, which are attributive to hyperactivity of fire evil and insufficiency of water, apply Cortex Phellodendri instead of Scutellariae to clear away the "prime-minister" fire and nourish kidney-yin.

Decoction of Five Drugs Containing
Astragali seu Hedysari and Cinnamomi
(Huangqi Guizhi Wuwu Tang)

INGREDIENTS:

Radix Astragali seu Hedysari	15 g
Radix Paeoniae Alba	10 g
Ramulus Cinnamomi	10 g
Rhizoma Zingiberis Recens	18 g
Fructus Ziziphi Jujubae	6 pcs

EFFICACY: Benefiting vital energy, regulating ying, activating yang-qi and relieving vessel obstruction; mainly for cases attributive to deficiency of qi, affection of wind and impediment of blood flow, which are manifested by numbness of muscles and skin, or pain in serious cases, pale tongue with white and smooth fur, unsmooth and tense or small and unsmooth, weak pulse.

INDICATIONS: 1. For cases of stroke manifested by hemiplegia, stiffness of tongue, aphasia, salivation, white and smooth fur on the tongue, slow and large pulse, which are attributive to declination of qi and blood and obstruction of meridians. 2. For cases with flaccidity and atrophy of limbs, pale tongue, sunken and weak pulse, which are attributive to impairment of qi and blood, and impediment of blood circulation, add Colla Cornus Cervi. 3. Applicable to cases of cerebral accidents, poliomyelitis, Guillain-Barre syndrome and progressive muscular dystrophy, marked by numbness of muscles and skin, flaccidity of limbs, or hemiplegia, which are attributive to declination of qi and blood and impediment of blood circulation.

INTERPRETATION: In sum, this prescription aims at benefiting qi and promoting blood circulation. The obstruction of blood vessels may be relieved when the qi is sufficient and the blood circulation is activated.

Decoction of Gentianae Macrophyllae
(Da Qinjiao Tang)

INGREDIENTS:

Radix Gentianae Macrophyllae	90 g
Radix Glycyrrhizae	60 g
Rhizoma Ligustici Chuanxiong	60 g
Radix Angelicae Sinensis	60 g
Radix Paeoniae Alba	60 g
Herba Asari	15 g
Rhizoma seu Radix Notopterygii	30 g
Radix Ledebouriellae	30 g
Radix Scutellariae	30 g
Gypsum Fibrosum	60 g
Radix Angelicae Dahuricae	30 g
Rhizoma Atractylodis Macrocephalae	30 g
Radix Rehmanniae	30 g
Radix Rehmanniae Praeparata	30 g
Poria	30 g
Radix Angelicae Pubescentis	60 g

All the above drugs are to be decocted in water for oral administration.

EFFICACY: Dispersing exopathic wind and clearing awaypathogenic heat.

INDICATIONS: Attacks of exopathic wind on the channels marked by numbness of muscles, skin, hands and feet, sudden deviation of the eye and mouth, rigidity of the extremities, failure to move the hands and feet, or accompanied by exterior syndrome of cold type or exterior syndrome of heat type marked by white tongue fur and floating pulse.

INTERPRETATION: Radix Gentianae Macrophyllae dispels exopathic wind to remove obstruction in the channels as a principal drug. Herba Asari, Rhizoma seu Radix Notopterygii, Radix Ledebouriellae, Radix Angelicae Dahuricae and Radix Angelicae Pubescentis, pungent in flavour and warmin nature, are used as assistant drugs to expel exopathic wind and other pathogens. Radix Angelicae Sinensis, Radix Paeoniae Alba and Radix Rehmanniae Praeparata nourish the blood and strengthen the muscles and tendon, expel pathogenic wind without impairing body fluid; Rhizoma Ligustici Chuanxiong reinforces the effects of Radix Angelicae Sinensis and Radix Paeoniae Alba in promoting blood flow and activating the channels; Rhizoma Atractylodis Macrocephalae and Poria replenish qi and invigorate the spleen to support the source of growth and the development of qi and blood. Radix Scutellariae, Gypsum Fibrosum and Radix Rehmanniae clear away pathogenic heat from the blood. All the drugs mentioned above are used as adjuvant drugs.

CAUTIONS: The recipe is contraindicated for cases with convulsion due to endogenous wind.

Decoction of Glycyrrhizae, Tritici Levis and Ziziphi Jujubae (Gancao Xiaomai Dazao Tang)

INGREDIENTS:

Radix Glycyrrhizae	15 g
Semen Tritici Levis	30 g
Fructus Ziziphi Jujubae	10 pcs

EFFICACY: Nourishing the heart and tranquilizing, regulating the middle jiao and soothe mental tension; mainly for hysteria manifested by lack of control over acts and emotions, anxiety, frequent yawning, reddish tongue without fur, small and rapid pulse.

INDICATIONS: 1. It is more effective when Radix Ophiopogonis and Radix Paeoniae Alba are added, since the former can calm the mental state and nourish yin, and the latter can nourish and soften the liver. 2. For cases of marked deficiency of heart-yin with vexation and constipation, add Bulbus Lilii and Semen Biotae to nourish the heart, calm the mental state, moisten the dryness evil and promote the bowel movement; for cases accompanied with insufficency of kidney-qi and frequent yawning, add Fructus Corni and Fructus Schisandrae to invigorate the kidney and strengthen the vital energy. 3. Also applicable to cases of manopause and other mental disorders with lack of control over acts and emotions, as well as cases of neurasthenia and cardiasthenia with palpitation, insomnia and vexation which are attributed to insufficiency of heart-yin.

Decoction of Nine Ingredients
Containing Notopterygii
(Jiu Wei Qianghuo Tang)

INGREDIENTS:

Rhizoma seu Radix Notopterygii	9 g
Radix Ledebouriellae	9 g
Rhizoma Atractylodis	9 g
Rhizoma LIgustici Chuanxiong	6 g
Radix Angelicae Dahuricae	6 g
Radix Rehmanniae	6 g
Radix Scutellariae	6 g
Herba Asari	3 g
Radix Glycyrrhizae	3 g

EFFICACY: Inducing sweating, expelling cold evil, eliminating wind evil and dampness evil and clearing away internal heat evil; mainly for cases caused by the attack of exogenous wind, cold and dampness evils, manifested by chilliness, fever, anhidrosis, headache, general aching, bitter mouth, thirst, whitish fur on the tongue, floating pulse, etc..

INDICATIONS: 1. For cases with feeling of fullness over the chest and epigastrium, nausea and greasy fur, attributive to severe stagnation of dampness evil omit Rehmanniae and Glycyrrhizae and add Caulis Perillae and Herba Agastachis to eliminate dampness evil; for cases with dry throat or sore throat omit Asari and add Herba Menthae to ease the throat; for cases without bitter mouth and thirst, decrease the dosage of Rehmanniae and Scutellariae. 2. Applicable to cases of toothache with wind-cold-superficies syndrome such as chilliness, headache, etc.. 3. Applicable to cases of trigeminal neuralgia, influenza, rheumatic arthritis, etc. with chilliness and headache, or toothache, or general aching, attributive to wind, cold and dampness evil located at the superficies with heat evil in the interior.

Decoction of Notopterygii
for Expelling Dampness
(Qianghuo Sheng Shi Tang)

INGREDIENTS:

Rhizoma seu Radix Notopterygii	9 g
Radix Angelicae Pubescentis	9 g
Rhizoma Ligustici	5 g
Radix Ledebouriellae	5 g
Rhizoma Ligustici Chuanxiong	5 g
Fructus Viticis	3 g
Radix Glycyrrhizae Praeparata	3 g

EFFICACY: Expelling wind and dampness evil; mainly for cases with wind-dampness evil located at the superficies, which are manifested by headache, heaviness over the head, general aching, chilliness, fever, whitish fur on the tongue, floating pulse.

INDICATIONS: 1. For lumbago attributive to the attack of cold-dampness, add Radix Stephaniae Tetrandrae, Radix Aconiti Praeparata or Radix Aconiti to warm yang-qi and meridians, and expel dampness and cold evil. 2. For cases of nasosinusitis manifested by stuffy nose, nasal discharge, headache, which attributive to the attack of exogenous wind-dampness, add Furctus Xanthii. 3. Also Applicable to cases of influenza, rheumatic arthritis, neurogenic headache, allergic, etc., which are attributive to the wind-dampness located at the superficies.

Decoction of Paeoniae and Glycyrrhizae
(Shaoyao Gancao Tang)

INGREDIENTS:

Radix Paeoniae Alba	24 g
Radix Glycyrrhizae Praeparata	12 g

EFFICACY: Benefiting yin, soothing the liver, relaxing spasm and relieving pain; mainly for cases attributive to insufficiency of ying-yin and conflict between the liver and spleen, which manifest abdominal colicky pain without change appetite, urination and defecation, reddish tongue with yellowish fur, wiry and rapid pulse or small and rapid pulse.

INDICATIONS: 1. The proportion of dosage between Paeoniae Alba and Glycyrrhizae is two to one. They are applied in large dose and the dosage of Paeoniae Alba may be as large as 30 g, or even 40 g. 2. Applicable to cases of dysmenorrhea attributive to insufficiency of ying-yin and dysfunction of liver-energy, which is accompanied by lower abdominal pain with desire of defecation, reddish tongue with yellowish fur, wiry and rapid pulse. 3. Also indicated for muscular spasm with reddish tongue, thin and white fur, small and wiry pulse, which are attributive to insufficiency of liver-blood and failure of nourishing the muscles. 4. Applicable to cases of irritable colon, neurasthenia, etc. marked by abdominal pain, which are attributive to insufficiency of ying-yin and dysfunction of liver-qi.

Decoction of Pinellia,
Atractylodis Macrocephalae and Gastrodiae
(Banxia Baizhu Tianma Tang)

INGREDIENTS:

Rhizoma Pinelliae	10 g
Rhizoma Gastrodiae	10 g
Poria	10 g
Rhizoma Atractylodis Macrocephalae	12 g
Exocarpium Citri Grandis	6 g
Radix Glycyrrhizae	2 g
Rhizoma Zingiberis Recens	3 pcs
Fructus Ziziphi Jujubae	2 pcs

EFFICACY: Dispersing phlegm, calming wind, strengthening the spleen and eliminating dampness; mainly for wind-phlegm syndrome attributive to production of phlegm by dampness in the spleen and the attack of endogenous liver-wind, which is manifested by dizziness, headache, heaviness of the head, feeling of oppression over the chest, nausea, vomiting, profuse expectoration of thick sputum, white and greasy fur on the tongue, wiry and smooth pulse, etc.

INDICATIONS: 1. For cases of stroke manifested by sudden onset of coma, lockjaw, salivation, white and greasy fur on the tongue, wiry and smooth pulse, which are attributive to obstruction of orifices by wind-phlegm, Bolus of Resina Liquidambaris Orientalis should be applied first and then followed by this prescription. In this case omit Glycyrrhizae and Ziziphi Jujubae, and add Rhizoma Arisaema cum Bile and Rhizoma Acori Graminei. 2. Applicable to cases of Meniere's syndrome, cerebral artherosclerosis, epilepsy, etc., marked by dizziness attributive to wind-phlegm.

Decoction of Pinelliae,
Atractylodis Macrocephalae and Gastrodiae (2)
(Banxia Baizhu Tianma Tang) (2)

INGREDIENTS:

Pinelliae	10 g
Fructus Hordei Germinatus	6 g
Massa Fermentata Medicinalis	6 g
Atractylodis Macrocephalae	12 g
Rhizoma Atractylodis	10 g
Radix Codonopsis Pilosulae	10 g
Radix Astragali seu Hedysari	6 g
Exocarpium Citri Grandis	6 g
Poria	10 g
Rhizoma Alismatis	6 g
Rhizoma Gastrodiae	10 g
Rhizoma Zingiberis	10 g
Cortex Phellodendri	10 g

EFFICACY: Dispersing phlegm, calming wind, strengthening the spleen and eliminating dampness.

INDICATIONS: Cases attributive to spleen hypofunction with production of phlegm and attack of endogenous liver-wind, which are manifested by headache, dizziness, cough with thick sputum, nausea and insomnia.

Decoction of Pinelliae
and Magnoliae Officinalis
(Banxia Houpo Tang)

INGREDIENTS:

Rhizoma Pinelliae	12 g
Cortex Magnoliae Officinalis	9 g
Poria	12 g
Rhizoma Zingiberis Recens	9 g
Folium Perillae	6 g

All the above drugs are to be decocted in water for oral administration.

EFFICACY: Promoting the circulation of qi to alleviate mental depression, lowering the adverse flow of qi and resolving phlegm.

INDICATIONS: Globus hystericus marked by a subjective sensation as if a plum pit is stuck in the throat which can neither be thrown up nor swallowed down, or accompanied by fullness and distress in the chest and hypochondrium, or cough or vomiting, white, moist or greasy fur of the tongue, and slippery or taut pulse.

Pharyngoneurosis, pharyngitis, edema of plica vocalis, bronchitis, bronchial asthma, neurogenic vomiting, gastric neurosis and vomiting of pregnancy marked by stagnancy of phlegm and qi or reversed flow of qi can be treated by the modified recipe.

Decoction of Poria for Eliminating Fluid
(Dao Shui Fuling Tang)

INGREDIENTS:

Poria	20 g
Radix Ophiopogonis	10 g
Rhizoma Alismatis	10 g
Rhizoma Atractylodis Macrocephalae	10 g
Cortex Mori Radicis	10 g
Folium Perillae	10 g
Semen Arecae	10 g
Fructus Chaenomelis	10 g
Pericarpium Arecae	10 g
Pericarpium Citri Reticulatae	6 g
Fructus Amomi	3 g
Radix Aucklandiae	3 g
Medulla Junci	5 bunches

EFFICACY: Promoting the circulation of vital energy, dispersing dampness, promoting diuresis and relieving edema; mainly for cases attributive to retention of fliud involving the lung, which are manifested by general pitted edema, dyspnea, orthopnea, anorexia, oliguria, white and thick fur on the tongue, and slow pulse.

INDICATIONS: 1. Applicable to cases with abdominal flatulence and pain, white and thick fur on the tongue and wiry pulse, which are attributive to the stagnation of vital energy and phlegm. 2. Applicable to cases of cirrhotic ascite, chronic nephritis, acute nephritis, etc. marked by edema, which are attributive to accumulation of fluid involving the lung; and to cases of chronic cholecystitis, duodenal ulcer, gastrointestinal neurosis, etc. marked by abdominal fullness and pain, which are attributive to stagnation of vital energy and phlegm.

Decoction of Seven Fine Drugs for Malaria
(Jie Nie Qi Bao Yin)

INGREDIENTS:

Radix dichroae	6 g
Cortex Magnoliae Officinalis	5 g
Semen Arecae	5 g
Fructus Tsaoko	5 g
Pericarpium Citri Reticulatae Viride	3 g
Exocarpium Citri Grandis	3 g
Radix Glycyrrhizae Praeparata	3 g
rice wine	q.s.

EFFICACY: Treating malaria, eliminating phlegm, regulating vital energy, expelling dampness evil; mainly for cases of chronic malaria with white and greasy fur on the tongue, wiry and smooth pulse, and strong physique, which are attributive to accumulation of phlegm-dampness.

INDICATIONS: 1. Applicable to cases of depressive psychosis manifested by dementia, incoherent speaking, emotional upset, profuse expectoration, feeling of oppression over the chest, white and greasy fur on the tongue, wiry and smooth pulse, which are attributive to involvement of mentality by phlegm. 2. Applicable to cases of cerebral malaria, arteriosclerotic psychosis and schizophrenia attributive to accumulation of phlegm.

Decoction of Uncariae cum Uncis
(Gouteng Yin)

INGREDIENTS:

Ramulus Uncariae cum Uncis	12 g
Cornu Saigae Tataricae	6 g
Rhizoma Gastrodiae	6 g
Radix Pseudostellariae	6 g
Scorpio	3 pcs
Radix Glycyrrhizae	3 g

EFFICACY: Clearing away heat, suppressing wind, supporting healthy energy and expelling evil; mainly for acute cases of infants manifested as high fever, palpitation, convulsion, lockjaw, fixation of eyes, red or crimson tongue, rapid pulse, which are attributive to hyperactivity of heat with production of wind.

INDICATIONS: 1. Applicable to eclampsia of pregnancy with red and uncoated tongue, wiry and rapid pulse, which is attributive to upward attack of liver-yang. 2. Also indicated for cases with dizziness, flushed cheeks, which are attributive to attack of the orifices by hyperactive liver-fire. 3. Applicable to cases of common cold, malaria, etc. with high fever and convulsion attributive to hyperactivity of heat with production of wind; and to cases of hypertension, Meniere's syndrome, etc. with dizziness attributive to hyperactivity of liver-fire.

Decoction of Ziziphi Spinosae
(Suanzaoren Tang)

INGREDIENTS:

Semen Ziziphi Spinosae	15 g
Rhizoma Anemarrhenae	10 g
Poria	10 g
Rhizoma Ligustici Chuanxiong	6 g
Radix Glycyrrhizae	6 g

EFFICACY: Nourishing liver-blood, tranquilizing and clearing away asthenic heat; mainly for cases due to insufficiency of liver-blood and flaming up of asthenic fire, manifested by vexation, insomnia, palpitation, night sweat, dry throat and mouth, wiry or small and rapid pulse.

INDICATIONS: 1. For cases with light and dreamful sleep, pale tongue, wriy and small pulse due to deficiency of both heart and gallbladder, add Radix Codonopsis Pilosulae and Dens Draconis to benefit qi and calm the patient. 2. For cases due to hyperactivity of asthenic fire evil, manifested by irritability, insomnia, dry mouth and throat, wiry and rapid pulse, add Fructus Ligustri Lucidi and Herba Ecliptae to nourish yin and clear away heat evil. 3. For cases with profuse night sweat, add Fructus Schisandrae to calm mental state and stop sweating; for cases with severe palpitation, add Dens Draconis to tranquilize the mind. 4. Applicable to cases of neurasthenia and schizophrenia with irritability and insomnia caused by insufficiency of liver- blood and hyperactivity of asthenic fire.

Ease Powder
(Xiao Yao San)

INGREDIENTS:

Radix bupleuri	15 g
Radix Angelicae Sinensis	15 g
Radix Paeoniae Alba	15 g
Poria	15 g
Rhizoma Atractylodis Macrocephalae	15 g
Rhizoma Zingiberis Recens Praeparata	3 g
Herba Menthae	3 g
Radix Glycyrrhizae Praeparata	6 g

PROCESS: Grind the above drugs except ginger and peppermint into powder take 6 to 9 grams each time with a decoction in small amount of roasted ginger and peppermint.

EFFICACY: Soothing the liver disperse depressed qi, and invigorating the spleen to nourish the blood.

INDICATIONS: Stagnation of the liver-qi with deficiency of the blood marked by hypochondriac pain, headache, dizziness, bitter mouth, dry throat, mental weariness and poor appetite, or alternate attacks of chills and fever, or irregular menstruation, distension in the breast, light redness of the tongue, taut and feeble pulse. Patients with chronic hepatitis, pleuritis, chronic gastritis, neurosis, irregular menstruation marked by symptoms of stagnation of liver-qi with deficiency of the blood can be treated by the modified recipe.

Golden Lock Bolus for Keep Kidney Essence
(Jin Suo Gu Jing Wan)

INGREDIENTS:

Semen Astragali Complanati	30 g
Semen Euryales	30 g
Semen Nelumbinis	30 g
Stamen Nelumbinis	15 g
Os Draconis	20 g
Concha Ostreae	20 g

EFFICACY: Strengthening kidney essence and stopping nocturnal emission; mainly for cases with hypofunction of kidney, characterized by nocturnal emission, fatigue, sorenss of limbs, lumbago, tinnitus, pale tongue with whitish fur, small and weak pulse.

INDICATIONS: 1. Applicable to deficiency of both kidney-yin and yang. For cases with deficiency of kidney-yin predominantly, add Fructus Ligustri Lucidi and Fructus Rosae Laevigatae, while for those with deficiency of kidney-yang predominantly, add Fructus Psoraleae and Pulvis of Cornu Cervi. It is not suitable for nocturnal emission due to hyperactivity of "prime-minister" fire. 2. For cases of leukorrhagia with thin discharge, attributive to deficiency of spleen-yang and yin, omit Stamen Nelumbinis and add Poria and Rhizoma Atractylodis Macrocephalae (in large dosage) to invigorate the spleen and kidney. 3. Applicable to cases of neurasthenia with nocturnal emission, and cervicitis with leukorrhagia, which are attributive to hypofunction of kidney.

Jade Maid Decoction
(Yu Nu Jian)

INGREDIENTS:

Gypsum Fibrosum	30 g
Radix Rehmanniae Praeparata	20 g
Radix Ophiopogonis	15 g
Radix Achyranthis Bidentatae	15 g
Rhizoma Anemarrhenae	10 g

EFFICACY: Clearing away stomach-fire and noursihing kidney-yin; mainly for toothache and headache due to insufficiency of kidney-yin and flaming up of stomach-fire, with bleeding of gum, restlessness, thirst, dry and reddish tongue with yellowish and dry fur.

INDICATIONS: 1. For cases of hematemesis and epistaxis due to hyper-activity of stomach-fire without marked consumption of kidney-yin, the dosage of Achyranthis Bidentatae should be heavier, and Rehmanniae is used instead of Rehmanniae Praeparata. For cases with reddish and dry, or smooth and uncoated tongue attributive to insufficiency of stomach fluid, add Radix Adenophorae Strictae and Herba Dendrobii to nourish stomach-yin and promote the production of body fluid. 2. Applicable to cases of trigeminal neuralgia, stomatitis, peri-odontitis, glossitis, etc. with toothache or headache, and hyperthyroidism, dia-betes mellitus with extreme thirst, which are attributive to insufficiency of kid-ney-fluid and hyperactivity of stomach-fire.

Longevity Powder
(Gui Ling Ji)

INGREDIENTS:

    Radix Ginseng

    Cornu Cervi Pantotrichum

    Hippocampus

    Herba Cistanchis

    Semen Cuscutae

    Semen Astragali Complanati

    Fructus Psoraleae

    Radix Aconiti

    Lateralis Praeparata

    Herba Epimedii

INDICATIONS: Nourishing the kidney, strengthening yang and replenishing vital essence. Symptoms caused by decline of fire from the gate of life and deficiency of kidney essence, manifested by mental tiredness, cold pain in loin and abdomen, impotence and seminal emission, metrorrhagia and metrostaxis, leukorrhagia and sterility. It can be used to treat the above symptoms resulting from neurosis, chronic nephritis and menopausal syndrome in women.

Major Decoction for Purging Down Digestive Qi
(Da Cheng Qi Tang)

INGREDIENTS:

Radix et Rhizoma Rhei	12 g
Cortex Magnoliae Officinalis	15 g

Fructus Aurantii Immaturus   12 g

Natrii Sulphas   9 g

EFFICACY: Relieving heat accumulation by mild effect.

INDICATIONS: Mild cases of excess syndrome of yangming-fuorgan, manifested by delirium, tidal fever, constipation, distension and fullness in the chest and abdomen, yellow shriveled tongue coating, smooth and swift pulse as well as the onset of dysentery with distending abdominal pain or epigastric fullness, tenesmus.

CAUTIONS: 1. Being a drastic recipe, it must be administered with great care to those of general asthenia, or to those whose external syndrome has not been relieved or to those with absence of dry stool in gastrointestinal tract. 2. The drastic effect of this recipe is harmful to the stomach-qi. Thus, immediate withdrawal is indicated once the effect attained. Over- administration prohibited. 3. It is never administered for pregnant women.

Oral Liquid for Health
(Kang Bao Kou Fu Ye)

INGREDIENTS:

Lac Regis Apis

Radix Acanthopanacis Senticosi

Rhizoma Polygonati

Radix Astragali seu Hedysari

Fructus Crataegi

Fructus Lycii

Herba Epimedii

Radix Rehmanniae Praeparata

EFFICACY: Invigorating qi and the kidney, strengthening the spleen and regulating the stomach, and nourishing the heart to calm the mind.

INDICATIONS: Dizziness, tinnitus, diminution of vision, hypoacusis, insomnia, amnesia, loss of appetite, sore and aching loin and knees, palpitation, short breath. It is also effecíve for the' treatment of the seqauelae of apoplexy, cerebral hypofunction, coronary vascular diseases, alopecia and others.

Oral Liquid of Ginseng and Acanthopanax
(Liang Shen Jing)

INGREDIENTS:

Radix Ginseng

Cortex Acnthopanax Radicis

EFFICACY: Supplementing qi, nourishing the blood, and strengthening the body.

INDICATIONS: Neurosis, weakness after diseases, seniledebility, anorexia, dyspepsia.

Pill for Calming Mental State
(An Shen Ding Zhi Wan)

INGREDIENTS:

Radix Codonopsis Pilosulae	12 g
Poria	12 g
Lignum Pini	12 g
Dens Draconis	20 g
Radix Polygalae	6 g
Rhizoma Acori Graminei	6 g

EFFICACY: Nourishing heart, calming mental state, and keeping heart-fire and kidney-water in balance; mainly for cases attributive to insufficiency of heart-qi and imbalance between heart-fire and kidney-water, which are manifested by dreaminess, timidness, palpitation, insomnia, pale tongue, small and weak pulse.

INDICATIONS: 1. Applicable to cases after epileptic attack manifested by spiritlessness, palpitation, shortness of breath, anorexia, profuse expectoration, pale tongue with whitish fur, small and smooth pulse, which are attributive to insufficiency of heart-qi and stagnation of phlegm in the heart orifice. 2. Indicated for cases of nocturnal emission attributive to imbalance between heart-fire and kidney-water, which are accompanied with palpitation, dizziness, spiritlessness, fatigue, pale tongue with whitish fur on the tongue, small and weak pulse. 3. Applicable to cases of sinus bradycardia, atrioculoventricular block, sinus arrhythmia, vegetative nervous dysfunction, neurasthenia, etc. marked by palpitation, insomnia, or nocturnal emission, which are attributive to insufficiency of heart-qi and imbalance between heart-fire and kidney-water.

Pill for Cerebral Thrombosis
(Yi Nao Fu Jian Wan)

INGREDIENTS:
    Radix Notoginseng
    Stigma Croci
    Rhizoma Ligustici Chuanxiong

EFFICACY: Supplementing the brain and invigorating the vitality, relaxing the channels and collaterals, and promoting blood circulation to remove blood stasis, waking up the patients from unconsciousness by climinating phlegm.

INDICATIONS: Symptoms and signs caused by acute cerebral embolism and cerebral thrombosis such as facial paralysis, hemiplegia, involuntary drooling, retraction of the tongue and difficulty in speaking.

CAUTION: Contraindicated for pregnant women.

Pill for Eliminating Phlegm Evil
(Gun Tan Wan)

INGREDIENTS:

Radix et Rhizoma Rhei	240 g
Radix Scutellariae	240 g
Lignum Aquilariae Resinatum	15 g
Lapis Chloriti	30 g

EFFICACY: Purging fire and eliminating phlegm; mainly for cases of chronic phlegm-syndrome of sthenic heat type, manifested by mania with frigthening, or dyspneic cough with thick sputum, or feeling of oppression over the chest and epigastrium, or dizziness with profuse expectoration, constipation, yellow and thick, greasy fur on the tongue, smooth and rapid, strong pulse.

INDICATIONS: 1. This formula cannot be taken as decoction. 2. Applicable to cases of nasosinusitis manifested by stuffy nose, headache, turbid, foul, thick and yellow nasal discharge, yellow and greasy fur on the tongue, wiry and rapid pulse, which are attributive to the attack of phlegm-heat from the spleen and stomach to the nasal orifice. 3. Applicable to cases of chronic suppurative otitis media accompanied with deafness, tinnitus, yellow and greasy fur on the tongue, wiry and rapid pulse, which are attributive to the attack of dampness-heat of liver and gallbladder to the orifice. 4. Applicable to cases of schizophrenia-, manic-depressive psychosis, chronic bronchitis, emphysema, etc., which are attributive to chronic phlegm-syndrome of sthenic heat type.

Pill for Lubricating Intestine
(Run Chang Wan)

INGREDIENTS:

Radix Angelicae Sinensis	10 g

Rhizoma seu Radix Notoperygii	10 g
Radix et Rhizoma Rhei	10 g
Semen Persicae	10 g
Fructus Cannabis	30 g
Mel	30 g

EFFICACY: Activating blood circulation, expelling wind, lubricating intestines and promoting bowel movement; mainly for cases of constipation accompanied with dizziness, wiry and small, rapid pulse, which are attributive to involvement of the lung and the intestine by liver-wind and consumption of body fluid.

INDICATIONS: 1. Applicable to cases of constipation occuring at the initial stage of trauma of lumbar vertebrae, such as prolapse of lumbar intervertebral disc, compressed fracture of lumbar vertebra, etc.. 2. Applicable to sequelae of cerebrovascular accidents and hypertension with constipation attributive to attack of the lung by liver-wind.

Pill for Relieving Epilepsy
(Ding Xian Wan)

INGREDIENTS:

Rhizoma Gastrodiae	6 g
bulbus Fritillariae Cirhosae	6 g
Rhizoma Pinelliae	6 g
Poria	6 g
Lignum Pini Poriferum	6 g
Radix Salviae Miltiorrhizae	6 g
Radix Ophiopogonis	6 g
Rhizoma Arisaema cum Bile	3 g
Scorpio	3 g
Rhizoma Acori Graminei	3 g

Bombyx Batryticatus	3 g
Succinum	3 g
Exocarpium Citri Grandis	4 g
Radix Polygalae	4 g
Cinnabaris	2 g
Radix Glycyrrhizae	2 g
Succus Lophatheri	30 g
Succus Zingiberis	30 g

EFFICACY: Eliminating phlegm, resuscitating, tranquilizing, suppressing wind and relieving convulsion; mainly for cases of epilepsy with dizziness and feeling or oppression over the chest before the attack, sudden fainting, convulsive seizures, salivation, or even incontinence of urine and feces, greasy fur on the tongue, wiry and smooth pulse, which are attributive to obstruction of meridians and upper orifices by wind-phlegm.

INDICATIONS: 1. For cases of apoplexy with sudden onset of face distortion, dysphasia, numbness of the limbs, or even hemiplegia, rigidity of the extremities, white and greasy fur on the tongue, floating and smooth pulse, which are attributive to attack of wind-phlegm to the meridians, omit Cinnabaris and Succinum from this prescription. 2. Applicable to cases of tetanus with trismus, convulsion, rigidity of the neck, or even opisthotonos, greasy fur on the tongue, wiry and tense pulse, which are attributive to the attack of wind and obstruction of the meridians by phlegm.

Powder for Treating Face-Distortion
(Qian Zheng San)

INGREDIENTS:

Rhizoma Typhonii	10 g
Bombyx Batryticatus	10 g
Scorpio	6 g

Wine   q.s.

EFFICACY: Expelling wind, dispersing phlegm, dredging the passage of meridians and stopping convulsion; mainly for cases of apoplexy attributive to the obstruction of meridians of the head by wind-phlegm, which are manifested by facial paralysis and distortion, or muscular twitching of the face, and smooth fur on the tongue, wiry pulse.

INDICATIONS: 1. It is suirtable for cases attributive to wind-phlegm, especially cold-dampness. 2. Typhonii and Scorpio are poisonous, overdosage should be avoided. 3. Applicable to cases attributive to obstruction of meridians by wind-phlegm, which are manifested as pain and immobility of the shoulder, white and greasy fur on the tongue. 4. Also applicable to facial paralysis, chorea, trigeminal neuralgia, which are attributive to obstruction of meridians by wind-phlegm.

Pill of Cinnabaris for Tranquilizing
(Zhushan An Shen Wan)

INGREDIENTS:

Cinnabaris (ground into powder in water)	15 g
Rhizoma Coptidis	12 g
Radix Glycyrrhizae Praeparata	10 g
Radix Rehmanniae	10 g
Radix Angelicae Sinensis	10 g

EFFICACY: Clearing away heart-fire, tranquilizing and nourishing heart-yin; mainly for cases due to flamming up of heart-fire and damage of yin-blood, manifested by irritability, insomnia, dreaminess, severe palpitation, feeling of oppressionand hot sensation in the chest, red tongue and small, rapid pulse.

INDICATIONS: 1. Asthenic fire with tender and reddish tongue, and small, rapid and weak pulse, caused by asthenia fire evil. 2. Feeling of oppression over the chest, small and smooth pulse, accompanied with heat-phlegm syndrome; irritability, reddish tongue, smooth pulse and domination of heart-fire accompanied with phlegm-heat. 3. Applicable to cases of neurasthenia with palpitation, insomnia and mental depression, attributive to domination of heart-fire. 4. Cinnabaris is poisonous, the dosage of which should be under 2 g once a time, and it should not be taken continuously for more than one week.

Pill of Margarita
(Zhenzhumu Wan)

INGREDIENTS:

Margarita	25 g
Os Draconis	20 g
Radix Rehmanniae Praeparata	20 g
Radix Angelicae Sinensis	12 g
Radix Codonopsis Pilosulae	12 g
Semen Ziziphi Spinosae	12 g
Semen Biotae	12 g
Lignum Pini Poriaferum	12 g
Cornu Rhinocerotis	3 g
Lignum Aquilariae Resinatum	6 g
Cinnabaris	1 g

EFFICACY: Nourishing yin, calming mental state and relieving palpitation; mainly for cases attributive to insufficiency of liver-blood and instability of mental state, manifested by insomnia, palpitation, dizziness, pale complexion, small and weak pulse.

INDICATIONS: Applicable to cases of sinus tachycardia, paroxysmal supraventricular tachycardia, auriculo-ventricular block, sinus arrhythmia, vegetative nervous dysfunction, neurasthenia, etc. marked by palpitation or insomnia, which are attributive to insufficiency of liver-blood and instability of mental state.

Pill of Poria
(Zhi Mi Fuling Wan)

INGREDIENTS:

Rhizoma Pinelliae	12 g
Poria	15 g
Fructus Aurantii	10 g
Natrii Sulfas	6 g
Succus Zingiberis	q.s.

EFFICACY: Drying dampness, promoting circulation of qi, expelling stubborn phlegm; mainly for cases attributive to retention of phlegm in the limbs, manifested by soreness over the arms which is more severe at night, flaccidity of the upper limbs, limited movement of the shoulder joint, white and greasy fur, sunken and smooth pulse, etc..

INDICATIONS: 1. Applicable to cases of dizziness accompanied with heaviness of the head, feeling of oppression over the chest, nausea, anorexia, somnolence, white and greasy fur on the tongue, sunken and smooth pulse, which are attributive to the failure of spleen to eliminate dampness and the attack of phlegm-dampness to lucid yang. 2. Also indicated for depressive psychosis attributive to obstruction of the heart by phlegm-dampness, which is manifested by dementia, silence or muttering to oneself, emotional upset, anorexia, white and greasy fur on the tongue, wiry and smooth pulse. 3. Also applicable to cases of rheumatoid arthritis, Meniere's syndrome, cerebral arteriosclerosis, schizophrenia, hysteria, etc., which are attributive to the attack of phlegm.

Powder of Ligustici Chuanxiong
Mixed with Camelliae Sinensis
(Chuanxiong Cha Tiao San)

INGREDIENTS:

Rhizoma Ligustic Chuanxiong	10 g
Herba Schizonepetae	10 g
Radix Angelicae Dahuricae	10 g
Rhizoma seu Radix Notopterygii	10 g
Radix Ledebouriellae	10 g
Herba Asari	3 g
Radix Glycyrrhizae	3 g
Folium Menthae	3 g
Folium Camelliae Sinensis	3 g

EFFICACY: Expelling wind evil and relieving pain; mainly for affection of exogenous wind evil, manifested as lingering headache which is bilateral or u-nilateral, or vertical, chilliness, fever, dizziness, stuffy nose, thin and white fur on the tongue and floating pulse.

INDICATIONS: Applicable to neurotic headache, acute nasosinusitis, common cold, etc., marked by headache, which are attributive to the attack of endogenous or exogenous wind.

Powder of Lilii and Talcum
(Baihe Huashi San)

INGREDIENTS:

Bulbus Lilii Praeparata	15 g

Talcum   30 g
   EFFICACY: Nourishing lung-yin, tranquilizing, clearing away interior-
heat and promoting diuresis; mainly for "Lilii" syndrome (depressive state of
psychic disease), manifested by mental disorder, irritability, insomnia, anorexi-
a, neither cold nor fever, bitter taste in the mouth, yellow urine, small, smooth
and rapid pulse, which is attributive to deficiency of heart-and lung-yin.
   INDICATIONS: Applicable to cases of neurasthenia and symptomatic psychosis, which are attributive to deficiency of heart-yin and lung-yin.

Powder of Oŏtheca Mantidis
(Sangpiaoxiao San)

INGREDIENTS:

Oŏtheca Mantidis	15 g
Lignum Pini Poriaferum	15 g
Os Draconis	20 g
Plastrum Testudinis	20 g
Radix Codonopsis Pilosulae	10 g
Radix Angelicae Sinensis	10 g
Radix Polygalae	6 g
Rhizoma Acori Graminei	6 g

   EFFICACY: Regulating and invigorating heart and kidney, stopping
spermatorrhoea; mainly for cases attributed to hypofunction of both heart and
kidney, which are manifested by frequent micturition, enuresis, nocturnal emission, trance, insomnia, amnesia, pale tongue with whitish fur, small and weak
pulse.
   INDICATIONS: For the aged with dripping urination (in the day) due to
hypofunction of kidney. Applicable to cases of neurasthenia, which is attributive
to hypofunction of both heart and kidney.

Powder of Pedicellus Melo
(Guadi San)

INGREDIENTS:

Pedicellus Melo	2 g
Semen Phaseoli	2 g
Semen Sojae Praeparatum	9 g

EFFICACY: Inducing vomiting and relieving stagnation of phlegm and food; mainly for cases attributive to retention of phlegm or food in the epigastrium.

INDICATIONS: Applicable to cases of epilepsy, schizophrenia, manic-depressive psychosis, etc. which are attributive to hyperactivity of sthenic evil.

Restorative Bolus with Tremendous Powder
(Hui Tian Zai Zao Wan)

INGREDIENTS:

Radix Ginseng

Calculus Bovis

Moschus

Os Tigris

Rhizoma Gastrodiae

Resina Draconis

Cornu Rhinocerotis

Sanguis Naemorhedi

EFFICACY: Dispelling wind, resolving phlegm and promoting blood circulation to remove obstruction in the channels.

INDICATIONS: Hemiplegia, facial hemiparalysis, soreness inthe loin and legs, numbness of limbs.

Sedative and Heart-Invigorating Pill
(An Shen Bu Xin Wan)

INGREDIENTS:
  Radix Salviae Miltiorrhizae
  Fructus Schisandrae
  Rhizoma Acori Graminei
  Emplastrium Sedativi
EFFICACY: Tranquilizing the mind and nourishing the heart.
INDICATIONS: Neurosis manifested by insomnia, amnesia, dizziness, tinnitus, palpitation.

Shi Guodong's Prescription
for Preparing Medicated Wine
(Shi Guodong Yin Jiu Fang)

INGREDIENTS:

Radix Angelicae Sinensis	10 g
Rhizoma seu Radix Notopterygii	10 g
Rhizoma Dioscoreae hypoglaucae	10 g
Radix Ledebouriellae	10 g
Radix Gentianae Macrophyllae	10 g
Radix Cyathulae	10 g
Nodus Pini	10 g
Fructus Lycii	10 g
Excrementum Bombycis	12 g
Carapax Trionycis Praeparata	15 g

Radix Solani	15 g
Os Tigris	6 g

INDICATIONS: 1. Applicable to cases of apoplexy with distortion of face, dysphasia, or hemiplegia, rigidity of limbs, tinnitus, dizziness, pale tongue with whitish fur, small and weak pulse, which are attributive to the deficiency of qi and blood and the attack of wind to the meridians. 2. Also indicated for cases of cold injury or chilblain with cold limbs, chilliness, numbness and weakness of limbs, fatigue, pale tongue with white and smooth fur, sunken and small pulse, which are attributive to accumulation of cold-dampness and impediment of blood circulation. 3. Also applicable to cases of rheumatic arthritis, sciatica, periomarthritis, tuberculosis of knees, etc. with arthralgia attributive to deficency of blood and attack of wind- dampness; and to cases of cerebrovascular accidents and multiple neuritis with limited mobility of limbs or even hemiplegia, which are attributive to deficiency of vital energy and blood and attack of wind.

Storax Pill
(Suhexiang Wan)

INGREDIENTS:

Resina Liquidambaris Orientalis	30 g
Moschus	60 g
Borneolum	30 g
Benzoinum	60 g
Radix Aristolochiae	60 g
Lignum Santali	60 g
Lignum Aquilariae Resinatum	60 g
Flos Caryophylli	60 g
Rhizoma Cyperi	60 g
Resina Olibani	30 g
Fructus Piperis Longi	60 g

Cornu Rhinocerotis	60 g
Cinnabaris	60 g
Rhizoma Atractylodis Macrocephalae	60 g
Fructus Chebulae	60 g

EFFICACY: Inducing resuscitation with aromatics, promoting the circulation of qi to relieve pain.

INDICATIONS: Cold syndrome of coma marked by sudden fainting, trismus, unconsciousness, or fullness with cold sensation in the chest and abdomen, nausea and so on. Cerebrovascular accident, hysterical syncope, psychogenic syncope, epilepsy, and concussion of brain during the stage of syncope marked by cold syndrome of coma can be treated with the recipe.

Tablet of Corydalis
Tuber for Alleviating Pain
(Yuahu Zhi Tong Pian)

INGREDIENTS:

Rhizoma Corydalis

Radix Angelicae Dahuricae

EFFICACY: Promoting blood circulation to remove blood stasis and regulating the flow of qi to alleviate pain.

INDICATIONS: Abdominalgia, stomachalgia, headache, dysmenorrhea, pain in the waist and lower extremities, hepatalgia, etc..

Tranquilizing Liver-Wind Decoction
(Zhen Gan Xi Feng Tang)

INGREDIENTS:

Radix Achyranthis Bidentatae	30 g
Ochra Haematitum	30 g
Os Draconis	20 g
Fossilia Ossis Mastodi	15 g
Concha Ostreae	15 g
Plastrum Testudinis	15 g
Radix Paconiae Alba	15 g
Radix Scrophulariae	15 g
Radix Asparagi	15 g
Fructus Meliae Toosendan	6 g
Fructus Hordei Germinatus	6 g
Herba Artemisiae Capillaris	6 g
Radix Glycyrrhizae	4 g

EFFICACY: Tranquilizing the liver to calm endogenous wind.

INDICATIONS: Syndrome of wind stirring inside due to excess of yang marked by vertigo, swollen eyes and tinnitus, pain and heat sensation in the head, or the limited sensation in the movement of limbs or wry mouth by degrees, or even falling down due to faintness, taut and forceful pulse. Cerebrovascular accident, hypertensive encephalopathy and so on marked by endogenous wind due to excess of yang can be treated by the modified recipe.

White Tiger Decoction
(Baihu Tang)

INGREDIENTS:

Gypsum Fibrosum	30 g
Rhizoma Anemarrhenae	9 g
Radix Glycyrrhizae Praeparata	3 g
Semen Oryzae Nonglutionosae	9 g

All the above drugs are to be decocted in water for oraladministration.

EFFICACY: Clearing away heat and promoting the production of body fluid.

INDICATIONS: Yangming channel diseases marked by high fever, flushed face, polydipsia, profuse perspiration, aversion to heat and full forceful pulse. It can be modified to treat influenza, epidemic encephalitis B, epidemic cerebrospinal meningitis, pneumonia and septicemia indicating excessive heat syndrome in the qi system.

Yougui Decoction
(You Gui Yin)

INGREDIENTS:

Radix Rehmanniae Praeparata	30 g
Rhizoma Dioscoreae	10 g
Fructus Corni	10 g
Cortex Eucommiae	10 g
Fructus Lycii	10 g
Radix Aconiti Praeparata	7 g

Cortex Cinnamomi   3 g

Radix Glycyrrhizae Praeparata   3 g

EFFICACY: Warming and invigorating kidney-yang; mainly for cases attributive to insufficency of kidney-yang, manifested by lumbago, cold limbs, shortness of breath, fatigue, impotence, nocturnal emission, pale tongue, small pulse, etc..

INDICATIONS: Applicable to cases of Addison's disease, Sheehan's disease, hypthyroidism, neurasthenia, etc., which are attributive to insufficiency of kidney-yang.

Yuzhen Powder
（Yu Zhen San）

INGREDIENTS:

Rhizoma Arisaematis   10 g

Radix Ledebouriellae   10 g

Radix Angelicae Dahuricae   10 g

Rhizoma Gastrodiae   10 g

Rhizoma seu Radix Notopterygii   10 g

Rhizoma Typhonii   10 g

Wine   q. s.

EFFICACY: Expelling wind evil, dispersing phlegm and stopping convulsion; mainly for tetanus.

INDICATIONS: It is only indicated for those cases when the body fluid and vital energy are not yet consumed. Also applicable to cases of headache accompanied with dizziness, insomnia, vomiting, white and moist fur on the tongue, wiry and smooth pulse, which are attributive to upward attack of wind-phlegm.

图书在版编目(CIP)数据

中医治疗精神－神经疾病:英文.侯景伦主编;李国华译.
－北京:学苑出版社,1996.5
ISBN 7－5077－1182－X

Ⅰ.中… Ⅱ.①侯… ②李…
Ⅲ.①精神病－中医疗法－英文 ②神经系统疾病－中医疗法－英文 Ⅳ.R.277.7

中国版本图书馆 CIP 数据核字(96)第 07830 号

中医治疗精神－神经疾病

主编　侯景伦

编委　赵　昕　耿春娥　李国华

学苑出版社出版
(中国北京万寿路西街11号)
邮政编码 100036
北京大兴沙窝店印刷厂印刷
中国国际图书贸易总公司发行
(中国北京车公庄西路35号)
北京邮政信箱第399号　邮政编码 100044
英文版　16 开本
1996 年 5 月第一版第一次印刷
ISBN 7－5077－1182－X/R·207

08100
14－E－3051P